MW01234987

The Grillers Cookbook

Different Grilling and Frying Recipes That Would Help Boost Your Body Health

By

Ralph Lehmann

The trademarks that are used are without any consent, and the publication of the trademark is without permission or backing by the trademark owner. All trademarks and brands within this book are for clarifying purposes only and are the owned by the owners themselves, not affiliated with this document.

Introduction

Thank you for purchasing the book, '365 Air Fryer Recipes'.

A lot of people across the world love fried food and will do just about anything to get their hands on it. People who hate cooking too manage to quickly fry these foods out of their freezer and satiate their taste buds. However, its no surprise that these fried foods come with a host of health related issues, thanks to the copious amounts of oil they soak in while getting fried.

To satiate your taste buds for fried foods without the health related side effects, you could use an air fryer. This technology uses way less oil compared to traditional deep-frying and is a much healthier but equally tasty option.

This book contains 365 air fried food recipes that will make your mouth water. You will find that you can eat French fries and any other fried foods without feeling any guilt at all. There are recipes for desserts in the book too! The recipes shared here will leave you craving for more. So without any further delay, lets get cooking.

Chapter 1: Non – Vegetarian Starters and Mains

Ingredients:

1.   Pork Burger Cutlets

½ lb. pork (Make sure that you mince the pork fine)

½ cup breadcrumbs

A pinch of salt to taste

¼ tsp. ginger finely chopped 1 green chili finely chopped 1 tsp. lemon juice

1 tbsp. fresh coriander leaves. Chop them finely

¼ tsp. red chili powder

½ cup of boiled peas

¼ tsp. cumin powder

¼ tsp. dried mango powder

Method:

Take a container and into it pour all the masalas, onions, green chilies, peas, coriander leaves, lemon juice, and ginger and 1-2 tbsp. breadcrumbs. Add the minced pork as well. Mix all the ingredients well.

Mold the mixture into round Cutlets. Press them gently. Now roll them out carefully.

Pre heat the Air Fryer at 250 Fahrenheit for 5 minutes. Open the basket of the Fryer and arrange the Cutlets in the basket. Close it carefully. Keep the fryer at 150 degrees for around 10 or 12 minutes. In between the cooking process, turn the Cutlets over to get auniform cook. Serve hot with mint chutney.

2.   Prawn Momos

Ingredients: For dough:

1 ½ cup all-purpose flour

½ tsp. salt

5 tbsp. water

For filling:

2 cups minced prawn 2 tbsp. oil

2 tsp. ginger-garlic paste 2 tsp. soya sauce

2 tsp. vinegar

Method:

Knead the dough and cover it with plastic wrap and set aside. Next, cook the ingredients for the filling and try to ensure that the prawn is covered well with the sauce.

Roll the dough and cut it into a square. Place the filling in the center. Now, wrap the dough to cover the filling and pinch the edges together.

Pre heat the Air fryer at 200° F for 5 minutes. Place the wontons in the fry basket and close it. Let them cook at the same temperature for another 20 minutes. Recommended sides are chili sauce or ketchup.

1   lb. boneless lamb cut into fingers 2 cup dry breadcrumbs

2   tsp. oregano

2 tsp. red chili flakes

Marinade:

1   ½ tbsp. ginger-garlic paste 4 tbsp. lemon juice

2   tsp. salt

1 tsp. pepper powder 1 tsp. red chili powder 6 tbsp. corn flour

4 eggs

Method:

Mix all the ingredients for the marinade and put the lamb fingers inside and let it rest overnight.

Mix the breadcrumbs, oregano and red chili flakes well and place the marinated fingers on this mixture. Cover it with plastic wrap and leave it till right before you serve to cook.

Pre heat the Air fryer at 160 degrees Fahrenheit for 5 minutes. Place the fingers in the fry basket and close it. Let them cook at the same temperature for another 15 minutes or so. Toss the fingers well so that they are cooked uniformly.

1   lb. boneless venison cut into fingers 2 cup dry breadcrumbs

2   tsp. oregano

2 tsp. red chili flakes 2 tsp. garlic paste Marinade:

1   ½ tbsp. ginger-garlic paste 4 tbsp. lemon juice

2   tsp. salt

1 tsp. red chili powder 6 tbsp. corn flour

4 eggs

Method:

Mix all the ingredients for the marinade and put the venison fingers inside and let it rest overnight.

Mix the breadcrumbs, oregano and red chili flakes well and place the marinated fingers on this mixture. Cover it with plastic wrap and leave it till right before you serve to cook.

Pre heat the Air fryer at 160 degrees Fahrenheit for 5 minutes. Place the fingers in the fry basket and close it. Let them cook at the same temperature for another 15 minutes or so. Toss the fingers well so that they are cooked uniformly. Drizzle the garlic paste and serve.

2 slices of white bread 1 tbsp. softened butter

½ lb. cut pork (Get the meat cut into cubes) 1 small capsicum

For Barbeque Sauce:

¼ tbsp. Worcestershire sauce

½ tsp. olive oil

½ flake garlic crushed

¼ cup chopped onion

¼ tsp. mustard powder

½ tbsp. sugar

¼ tbsp. red chili sauce 1 tbsp. tomato ketchup

½ cup water.

A pinch of salt and black pepper to taste

Method:

Take the slices of bread and remove the edges. Now cut the slices horizontally.

Cook the ingredients for the sauce and wait till it thickens. Now, add the pork to the sauce and stir till it obtains the flavors. Roast the capsicum and peel the skin off. Cut the capsicum into slices. Mix the ingredients together and apply it to the bread slices.

Pre-heat the Air Fryer for 5 minutes at 300 Fahrenheit. Open the basket of the Fryer and place the prepared sandwiches in it such that no two sandwiches are touching each other. Now keep the fryer at 250 degrees for around 15 minutes. Turn the sandwiches in between the cooking process to cook both slices. Serve the sandwiches with tomato ketchup or mint chutney.

1   lb. lamb (Cut into cubes) 2 ½ tsp. ginger-garlic paste 1 tsp. red chili sauce

¼ tsp. salt

¼ tsp. red chili powder/black pepper

A few drops of edible orange food coloring

For sauce:

2   tbsp. olive oil

1 ½ tsp. ginger garlic paste

½ tbsp. red chili sauce 2 tbsp. tomato ketchup 2 tsp. soya sauce

1-2 tbsp. honey

¼ tsp. Ajinomoto

1-2 tsp. red chili flakes

Method:

Mix all the ingredients for the marinade and put the lamb cubes inside and let it rest overnight.

Mix the breadcrumbs, oregano and red chili flakes well and place the marinated fingers on this mixture. Cover it with plastic wrap and leave it till right before you serve to cook.

Pre heat the Air fryer at 160 degrees Fahrenheit for 5 minutes. Place the fingers in the fry basket and close it. Let them cook at the same temperature for another 15 minutes or so. Toss the fingers well so that they are cooked uniformly.

Ingredients:

7. Cheese Chicken Fries

1 lb. chicken (Cut in to long fingers)

Ingredients for the marinade:

1 tbsp. olive oil

1 tsp. mixed herbs

½ tsp. red chili flakes A pinch of salt to taste 1 tbsp. lemon juice

For the garnish:

1   cup melted cheddar cheese

Method:

Take all the ingredients mentioned under the heading "For the marinade" and mix them well.

Cook the chicken fingers and soak them in the marinade.

Pre heat the Air Fryer for around 5 minutes at 300 Fahrenheit. Take out the basket of the fryer and place the chicken fingers in them. Close the basket. Now keep the fryer at 220 Fahrenheit for 20 or 25 minutes. In between the process, toss the fries twice or thrice so that they get cooked properly.

Towards the end of the cooking process (the last 2 minutes or so), sprinkle the cut coriander leaves on the fries. Add the melted cheddar cheese over the fries and serve hot.

One pizza base

Grated pizza cheese (mozzarella cheese preferably) for topping Some pizza topping sauce

Use cooking oil for brushing and topping purposes

Ingredients for topping:

2   onions chopped

½ lb. chicken (Cut the chicken into tiny pieces) 2 capsicums chopped

2 tomatoes that have been deseeded and chopped 1 tbsp. (optional) mushrooms/corns

2 tsp. pizza seasoning

Some cottage cheese that has been cut into small cubes (optional)

Method:

Put the pizza base in a pre-heated Air fryer for around 5 minutes. (Pre heated to 340 Fahrenheit).

Take out the base. Pour some pizza sauce on top of the base at the center. Using a spoon spread the sauce over the base making sure that you leave some gap around the circumference. Grate some mozzarella cheese and sprinkle it over the sauce layer.

Take all the vegetables and the chicken mentioned in the ingredient list above and mix them in a bowl. Add some oil and seasoning. Also add some salt and pepper according to taste. Mix them properly. Put this topping over the layer of cheese on the pizza. Now sprinkle some more grated cheese and pizza seasoning on top of this layer.

Pre heat the Air Fryer at 250 Fahrenheit for around 5 minutes. Open the fry basket and place the pizza inside. Close the basket and keep the fryer at 170 degrees for another 10 minutes. If you feel that it is undercooked you may put it at the same temperature for another 2 minutes or so.

1   lb. boneless chicken breast cut into fingers 2 cup dry breadcrumbs

2   tsp. oregano

2 tsp. red chili flakes

Marinade:

1   ½ tbsp. ginger-garlic paste 4 tbsp. lemon juice

2   tsp. salt

1 tsp. pepper powder 1 tsp. red chili powder 6 tbsp. corn flour

4 eggs

Method:

Mix all the ingredients for the marinade and put the chicken fingers inside and let it rest overnight.

Mix the breadcrumbs, oregano and red chili flakes well and place the marinated fingers on this mixture. Cover it with plastic wrap and leave it till right before you serve to cook.

Pre heat the Air fryer at 160 degrees Fahrenheit for 5 minutes. Place the fingers in the fry basket and close it. Let them cook at the same temperature for another 15 minutes or so. Toss the fingers well so that they are cooked uniformly.

10. Venison Wontons

Ingredients: For dough:

1 ½ cup all-purpose flour

½ tsp. salt

5 tbsp. water

For filling:

2 cups minced venison 2 tbsp. oil

2 tsp. ginger-garlic paste 2 tsp. soya sauce

2 tsp. vinegar

Method:

Knead the dough and cover it with plastic wrap and set aside. Next, cook the ingredients for the filling and try to ensure that the venison is covered well with the sauce.

Roll the dough and place the filling in the center. Now, wrap the dough to cover the filling and pinch the edges together.

Pre heat the Air fryer at 200° F for 5 minutes. Place the wontons in the fry basket and close it. Let them cook at the same temperature for another 20 minutes. Recommended sides are chili sauce or ketchup.

Ingredients:

11.   Chicken Croquette

2   lb. boneless chicken cut into 1½" pieces

1st Marinade:

3   tbsp. vinegar or lemon juice 2 or 3 tsp. paprika

1 tsp. black pepper 1 tsp. salt

3 tsp. ginger-garlic paste

2nd Marinade:

1 cup yogurt

4 tsp. tandoori masala

2 tbsp. dry fenugreek leaves 1 tsp. black salt

1 tsp. chat masala

1 tsp. garam masala powder 1 tsp. red chili powder

1 tsp. salt

3 drops of red color

Method:

Make the first marinade and soak the cut chicken in it for four hours. While this is happening, make the second marinade and soak the chicken in it overnight to let the flavors blend.

Pre heat the Air fryer at 160 degrees Fahrenheit for 5 minutes. Place the fingers in the fry basket and close it. Let them cook at the same temperature for another 15 minutes or so. Toss the fingers well so that they are cooked uniformly. Serve them with mint chutney.

1   lb. veal (Cut into fingers) 2 ½ tsp. ginger-garlic paste 1 tsp. red chili sauce

¼ tsp. salt

¼ tsp. red chili powder/black pepper

A few drops of edible orange food coloring

For sauce:

2   tbsp. olive oil

1 ½ tsp. ginger garlic paste

½ tbsp. red chili sauce 2 tbsp. tomato ketchup 2 tsp. soya sauce

1-2 tbsp. honey

¼ tsp. Ajinomoto

1-2 tsp. red chili flakes

Method:

Mix all the ingredients for the marinade and put the veal fingers inside and let it rest overnight.

Mix the breadcrumbs, oregano and red chili flakes well and place the marinated fingers on this mixture. Cover it with plastic wrap and leave it till right before you serve to cook.

Pre heat the Air fryer at 160 degrees Fahrenheit for 5 minutes. Place the fingers in the fry basket and close it. Let them cook at the same temperature for another 15 minutes or so. Toss the fingers well so that they are cooked uniformly.

1 lb. boneless pork cubed 3 onions chopped

5 green chilies-roughly chopped 1 ½ tbsp. ginger paste

1 ½ tsp. garlic paste 1 ½ tsp. salt

3 tsp. lemon juice

2 tsp. garam masala

4 tbsp. chopped coriander 3 tbsp. cream

2 tbsp. coriander powder 4 tbsp. fresh mint chopped 3 tbsp. chopped capsicum 3 eggs

2 ½ tbsp. white sesame seeds

Method:

Mix the dry ingredients in a bowl. Make the mixture into a smooth paste and coat the pork cubes with the mixture. Beat the eggs in a bowl and add a little salt to them.

Dip the cubes in the egg mixture and coat them with sesame seeds and leave them in the refrigerator for an hour.

Pre heat the Air fryer at 290 Fahrenheit for around 5 minutes. Place the kebabs in the basket and let them cook for another 25 minutes at the same temperature. Turn the kebabs over in between the cooking process to get auniform cook. Serve the kebabs with mint chutney.

½ lb. minced veal

½ cup breadcrumbs

A pinch of salt to taste

¼ tsp. ginger finely chopped 1 green chili finely chopped 1 tsp. lemon juice

1 tbsp. fresh coriander leaves. Chop them finely

¼ tsp. red chili powder

½ cup of boiled peas

¼ tsp. cumin powder

¼ tsp. dried mango powder

Method:

Take a container and into it pour all the masalas, onions, green chilies, peas, coriander leaves, lemon juice, and ginger and 1-2 tbsp. breadcrumbs. Add the minced veal as well. Mix all the ingredients well.

Mold the mixture into round patties. Press them gently. Now roll them out carefully.

Pre heat the Air Fryer at 250 Fahrenheit for 5 minutes. Open the basket of the Fryer and arrange the patties in the basket. Close it carefully. Keep the fryer at 150 degrees for around 10 or 12 minutes. In between the cooking process, turn the patties over to get auniform cook. Serve hot with mint chutney.

15. Pork Wontons

Ingredients: For dough:

1 ½ cup all-purpose flour

½ tsp. salt

5 tbsp. water

For filling:

2 cups minced pork 2 tbsp. oil

2 tsp. ginger-garlic paste 2 tsp. soya sauce

2 tsp. vinegar

Method:

Knead the dough and cover it with plastic wrap and set aside. Next, cook the ingredients for the filling and try to ensure that the pork is covered well with the sauce.

Roll the dough and place the filling in the center. Now, wrap the dough to cover the filling and pinch the edges together.

Pre heat the Air fryer at 200° F for 5 minutes. Place the wontons in the fry basket and close it. Let them cook at the same temperature for another 20 minutes. Recommended sides are chili sauce or ketchup.

2 slices of white bread 1 tbsp. softened butter

½ lb. cubed veal 1 small capsicum

For Barbeque Sauce:

¼ tbsp. Worcestershire sauce

½ tsp. olive oil

½ flake garlic crushed

¼ cup chopped onion

¼ tsp. mustard powder

½ tbsp. sugar

¼ tbsp. red chili sauce

½ cup water

Method:

Take the slices of bread and remove the edges. Now cut the slices horizontally.

Cook the ingredients for the sauce and wait till it thickens. Now, add the veal to the sauce and stir till it obtains the flavors. Roast the capsicum and peel the skin off. Cut the capsicum into slices. Mix the ingredients together and apply it to the bread slices.

Pre-heat the Air Fryer for 5 minutes at 300 Fahrenheit. Open the basket of the Fryer and place the prepared sandwiches in it such that no two sandwiches are touching each other. Now keep the fryer at 250 degrees for around 15 minutes. Turn the sandwiches in between the cooking process to cook both slices. Serve the sandwiches with tomato ketchup or mint chutney.

2 cups sliced lamb

1 big capsicum (Cut this capsicum into big cubes)

1 onion (Cut it into quarters. Now separate the layers carefully.) 5 tbsp. gram flour

A pinch of salt to taste

For the filling:

2 cup fresh green coriander

½ cup mint leaves 4 tsp. fennel

2 tbsp. ginger-garlic paste 1 small onion

6-7 flakes garlic (optional) Salt to taste

3 tbsp. lemon juice

Method:

You will first need to make the chutney. Add the ingredients to a blender and make a thick paste. Slit the pieces of lamb and stuff half the paste into the cavity obtained.

Take the remaining paste and add it to the gram flour and salt. Toss the pieces of lamb in this mixture and set aside.

Apply a little bit of the mixture on the capsicum and onion. Place these on a stick along with the lamb pieces.

Pre heat the Air Fryer at 290 Fahrenheit for around 5 minutes. Open the basket. Arrange the satay sticks properly. Close the basket. Keep the sticks with the lamb at 180 degrees for around half an hour while the sticks with the vegetables are to be kept at the same temperature for only 7 minutes. Turn the sticks in between so that one side does not get burnt and also to provide a uniform cook.

18. Chili Cheese Pork

Ingredients: For pork fingers:

1 lb. pork (Cut in to long strips) 2 ½ tsp. ginger-garlic paste

1   tsp. red chili sauce

¼ tsp. salt

¼ tsp. red chili powder/black pepper

A few drops of edible orange food coloring

For sauce:

2   tbsp. olive oil

1 ½ tsp. ginger garlic paste

½ tbsp. red chili sauce 2 tbsp. tomato ketchup 2 tsp. soya sauce

1-2 tbsp. honey

¼ tsp. Ajinomoto

1-2 tsp. red chili flakes

Method:

Mix all the ingredients for the marinade and put the pork fingers inside and let it rest overnight.

Mix the breadcrumbs, oregano and red chili flakes well and place the marinated fingers on this mixture. Cover it with plastic wrap and leave it till right before you serve to cook.

Pre heat the Air fryer at 160 degrees Fahrenheit for 5 minutes. Place the fingers in the fry basket and close it. Let them cook at the same temperature for another 15 minutes or so. Toss the fingers well so that they are cooked uniformly.

1   lb. boneless beef steak cut into fingers 2 cup dry breadcrumbs

2   tsp. oregano

2 tsp. red chili flakes

Marinade:

1   ½ tbsp. ginger-garlic paste 4 tbsp. lemon juice

2   tsp. salt

1 tsp. pepper powder 1 tsp. red chili powder 6 tbsp. corn flour

4 eggs

Method:

Mix all the ingredients for the marinade and put the beef fingers inside and let it rest overnight.

Mix the breadcrumbs, oregano and red chili flakes well and place the marinated fingers on this mixture. Cover it with plastic wrap and leave it till right before you serve to cook.

Pre heat the Air fryer at 160 degrees Fahrenheit for 5 minutes. Place the fingers in the fry basket and close it. Let them cook at the same temperature for another 15 minutes or so. Toss the fingers well so that they are cooked uniformly.

2 slices of white bread 1 tbsp. softened butter 1 tin tuna

1 small capsicum

For Barbeque Sauce:

¼ tbsp. Worcestershire sauce

½ tsp. olive oil

½ flake garlic crushed

¼ cup chopped onion

¼ tsp. mustard powder

½ tbsp. sugar

¼ tbsp. red chili sauce 1 tbsp. tomato ketchup

½ cup water.

A pinch of salt and black pepper to taste

Method:

Take the slices of bread and remove the edges. Now cut the slices horizontally.

Cook the ingredients for the sauce and wait till it thickens. Now, add the fish to the sauce and stir till it obtains the flavors. Roast the capsicum and peel the skin off. Cut the capsicum into slices. Mix the ingredients together and apply it to the bread slices.

Pre-heat the Air Fryer for 5 minutes at 300 Fahrenheit. Open the basket of the Fryer and place the prepared sandwiches in it such that no two sandwiches are touching each other. Now keep the fryer at 250 degrees for around 15 minutes. Turn the sandwiches in between the cooking process to cook both slices. Serve the sandwiches with tomato ketchup or mint chutney.

1   lb. boneless mutton cut into fingers 2 cup dry breadcrumbs

2   tsp. oregano

2 tsp. red chili flakes

Marinade:

1   ½ tbsp. ginger-garlic paste 4 tbsp. lemon juice

2   tsp. salt

1 tsp. pepper powder 1 tsp. red chili powder 6 tbsp. corn flour

4 eggs

Method:

Mix all the ingredients for the marinade and put the mutton fingers inside and let it rest overnight.

Mix the breadcrumbs, oregano and red chili flakes well and place the marinated fingers on this mixture. Cover it with plastic wrap and leave it till right before you serve to cook.

Pre heat the Air fryer at 160 degrees Fahrenheit for 5 minutes. Place the fingers in the fry basket and close it. Let them cook at the same temperature for another 15 minutes or so. Toss the fingers well so that they are cooked uniformly.

1   lb. boneless pork cut into fingers 2 cup dry breadcrumbs

2   tsp. oregano

2 tsp. red chili flakes

Marinade:

1   ½ tbsp. ginger-garlic paste 4 tbsp. lemon juice

2   tsp. salt

1 tsp. pepper powder 1 tsp. red chili powder 6 tbsp. corn flour

4 eggs

Method:

Mix all the ingredients for the marinade and put the pork fingers inside and let it rest overnight.

Mix the breadcrumbs, oregano and red chili flakes well and place the marinated fingers on this mixture. Cover it with plastic wrap and leave it till right before you serve to cook.

Pre heat the Air fryer at 160 degrees Fahrenheit for 5 minutes. Place the fingers in the fry basket and close it. Let them cook at the same temperature for another 15 minutes or so. Toss the fingers well so that they are cooked uniformly.

1 lb. boneless beef liver (Chop into cubes) 3 onions chopped

5 green chilies-roughly chopped 1 ½ tbsp. ginger paste

1 ½ tsp. garlic paste 1 ½ tsp. salt

3 tsp. lemon juice

2 tsp. garam masala

4 tbsp. chopped coriander 3 tbsp. cream

2 tbsp. coriander powder

4 tbsp. fresh mint (chopped) 3 tbsp. chopped capsicum

2 tbsp. peanut flour 3 eggs

Method:

Mix the dry ingredients in a bowl. Make the mixture into a smooth paste and coat the beef cubes with the mixture. Beat the eggs in a bowl and add a little salt to them.

Dip the cubes in the egg mixture and coat them with sesame seeds and leave them in the refrigerator for an hour.

Pre heat the Air fryer at 290 Fahrenheit for around 5 minutes. Place the kebabs in the basket and let them cook for another 25 minutes at the same temperature. Turn the kebabs over in between the cooking process to get auniform cook. Serve the kebabs with mint chutney.

24. Beef Wontons

Ingredients: For dough:

1 ½ cup all-purpose flour

½ tsp. salt

5 tbsp. water

For filling:

2 cups minced beef steak 2 tbsp. oil

2 tsp. ginger-garlic paste 2 tsp. soya sauce

2 tsp. vinegar

Method:

Knead the dough and cover it with plastic wrap and set aside. Next, cook the ingredients for the filling and try to ensure that the beef is covered well with the sauce.

Roll the dough and place the filling in the center. Now, wrap the dough to cover the filling and pinch the edges together.

Pre heat the Air fryer at 200° F for 5 minutes. Place the wontons in the fry basket and close it. Let them cook at the same temperature for another 20 minutes. Recommended sides are chili sauce or ketchup.

25.   Lamb Tikka

Ingredients:

2 cups sliced lamb

1 big capsicum (Cut this capsicum into big cubes)

1   onion (Cut it into quarters. Now separate the layers carefully.) 5 tbsp. gram flour

A pinch of salt to taste

For the filling:

2   cup fresh green coriander

½ cup mint leaves 4 tsp. fennel

2   tbsp. ginger-garlic paste 1 small onion

6-7 flakes garlic

3   tbsp. lemon juice Salt to taste Method:

You will first need to make the chutney. Add the ingredients to a blender and make a thick paste. Slit the pieces of lamb and stuff half the paste into the cavity obtained.

Take the remaining paste and add it to the gram flour and salt. Toss the pieces of lamb in this mixture and set aside.

Apply a little bit of the mixture on the capsicum and onion. Place these on a stick along with the lamb pieces.

Pre heat the Air Fryer at 290 Fahrenheit for around 5 minutes. Open the basket. Arrange the satay sticks properly. Close the basket. Keep the sticks with the lamb at 180 degrees for around half an hour while the sticks with the vegetables are to be kept at the same temperature for only 7 minutes. Turn the sticks in between so that one side does not get burnt and also to provide a uniform cook.

26.   Prawn Samosa

Ingredients: For wrappers:

2 tbsp. unsalted butter

1 ½ cup all-purpose flour A pinch of salt to taste

Add as much water as required to make the dough stiff and firm

For filling:

1 lb. prawn

¼ cup boiled peas

1 tsp. powdered ginger

1 or 2 green chilies that are finely chopped or mashed

½ tsp. cumin

1   tsp. coarsely crushed coriander 1 dry red chili broken into pieces A small amount of salt (to taste)

½ tsp. dried mango powder

½ tsp. red chili power. 1-2 tbsp. coriander.

Method:

You will first need to make the outer covering. In a large bowl, add the flour, butter and enough water to knead it into dough that is stiff. Transfer this to a container and leave it to rest for five minutes.

Place a pan on medium flame and add the oil. Roast the mustard seeds and once roasted, add the coriander seeds and the chopped dry red chilies. Add all the dry ingredients for the filling and mix the ingredients well. Add a little water and continue to stir the ingredients.

Make small balls out of the dough and roll them out. Cut the rolled out dough into halves and apply a little water on the edges to help you fold the halves into a cone. Add the filling to the cone and close up the samosa.

Pre-heat the Air Fryer for around 5 to 6 minutes at 300 Fahrenheit. Place all the samosas in the fry basket and close the basket properly. Keep the Air Fryer at 200 degrees for another 20 to 25 minutes. Around the halfway point, open the basket and turn the samosas over for uniform cooking. After this, fry at 250 degrees for around 10 minutes in order to give them the desired golden brown color. Serve hot. Recommended sides are tamarind or mint chutney.

2   lb. chicken breasts cubed 3 onions chopped

5 green chilies-roughly chopped 1 ½ tbsp. ginger paste

1 ½ tsp. garlic paste 1 ½ tsp. salt

3 tsp. lemon juice

2 tsp. garam masala

4 tbsp. chopped coriander 3 tbsp. cream

2 tbsp. coriander powder

4 tbsp. fresh mint (chopped) 3 tbsp. chopped capsicum

2 tbsp. peanut flour 3 eggs

Method:

Mix the dry ingredients in a bowl. Make the mixture into a smooth paste and coat the chicken cubes with the mixture. Beat the eggs in a bowl and add a little salt to them.

Dip the cubes in the egg mixture and coat them with sesame seeds and leave them in the refrigerator for an hour.

Pre heat the Air fryer at 290 Fahrenheit for around 5 minutes. Place the kebabs in the basket and let them cook for another 25 minutes at the same temperature. Turn the kebabs over in between the cooking process to get auniform cook. Serve the kebabs with mint chutney.

2 lb. mutton chopped 3 onions chopped

5 green chilies-roughly chopped 1 ½ tbsp. ginger paste

1 ½ tsp. garlic paste 1 ½ tsp. salt

3 tsp. lemon juice

2 tsp. garam masala

4 tbsp. chopped coriander 3 tbsp. cream

2 tbsp. coriander powder

4 tbsp. fresh mint (chopped) 3 tbsp. chopped capsicum

2 tbsp. peanut flour 3 eggs

Method:

Mix the dry ingredients in a bowl. Make the mixture into a smooth paste and coat the mutton cubes with the mixture. Beat the eggs in a bowl and add a little salt to them.

Dip the cubes in the egg mixture and coat them with sesame seeds and leave them in the refrigerator for an hour.

Pre heat the Air fryer at 290 Fahrenheit for around 5 minutes. Place the kebabs in the basket and let them cook for another 25 minutes at the same temperature. Turn the kebabs over in between the cooking process to get auniform cook. Serve the kebabs with mint chutney.

2 cups minced chicken 2 tbsp. oil

2 tsp. ginger-garlic paste 2 tsp. soya sauce

2 tsp. vinegar

Method:

Knead the dough and cover it with plastic wrap and set aside. Next, cook the ingredients for the filling and try to ensure that the beef is covered well with the sauce.

Roll the dough and cut it into a square. Place the filling in the center. Now, wrap the dough to cover the filling and pinch the edges together.

Pre heat the Air fryer at 200° F for 5 minutes. Place the wontons in the fry basket and close it. Let them cook at the same temperature for another 20 minutes. Recommended sides are chili sauce or ketchup.

2 cups minced lamb 2 tbsp. oil

2 tsp. ginger-garlic paste 2 tsp. soya sauce

2 tsp. vinegar

Method:

Knead the dough and cover it with plastic wrap and set aside. Next, cook the ingredients for the filling and try to ensure that the lamb is covered well with the sauce.

Roll the dough and cut it into a square. Place the filling in the center. Now, wrap the dough to cover the filling and pinch the edges together.

Pre heat the Air fryer at 200° F for 5 minutes. Place the wontons in the fry basket and close it. Let them cook at the same temperature for another 20 minutes. Recommended sides are chili sauce or ketchup.

2 cups minced beef steak 2 tbsp. oil

2 tsp. ginger-garlic paste 2 tsp. soya sauce

2 tsp. vinegar

Method:

Knead the dough and cover it with plastic wrap and set aside. Next, cook the ingredients for the filling and try to ensure that the beef is covered well with the sauce.

Roll the dough and cut it into a square. Place the filling in the center. Now, wrap the dough to cover the filling and pinch the edges together.

Pre heat the Air fryer at 200° F for 5 minutes. Place the wontons in the fry basket and close it. Let them cook at the same temperature for another 20 minutes. Recommended sides are chili sauce or ketchup.

2 cups sliced chicken

1 big capsicum (Cut this capsicum into big cubes)

1   onion (Cut it into quarters. Now separate the layers carefully.) 5 tbsp. gram flour

A pinch of salt to taste

For the filling:

2   cup fresh green coriander

½ cup mint leaves 4 tsp. fennel

2   tbsp. ginger-garlic paste 1 small onion

6-7 flakes garlic (optional) Salt to taste

3   tbsp. lemon juice

Method:

You will first need to make the chutney. Add the ingredients to a blender and make a thick paste. Slit the pieces of chicken and stuff half the paste into the cavity obtained.

Take the remaining paste and add it to the gram flour and salt. Toss the pieces of chicken in this mixture and set aside.

Apply a little bit of the mixture on the capsicum and onion. Place these on a stick along with the chicken pieces.

Pre heat the Air Fryer at 290 Fahrenheit for around 5 minutes. Open the basket. Arrange the satay sticks properly. Close the basket. Keep the sticks with the chicken at 180 degrees for around half an hour while the sticks with the vegetables are to be kept at the same temperature for only 7 minutes. Turn the sticks in between so that one side does not get burnt and also to provide a uniform cook.

2 cups sliced pork belly

1 big capsicum (Cut this capsicum into big cubes)

1   onion (Cut it into quarters. Now separate the layers carefully.) 5 tbsp. gram flour

A pinch of salt to taste

For the filling:

2   cup fresh green coriander

½ cup mint leaves 4 tsp. fennel

2   tbsp. ginger-garlic paste 1 small onion

6-7 flakes garlic (optional) Salt to taste

3   tbsp. lemon juice

Method:

You will first need to make the chutney. Add the ingredients to a blender and make a thick paste. Slit the pieces of pork and stuff half the paste into the cavity obtained.

Take the remaining paste and add it to the gram flour and salt. Toss the pieces of Pork in this mixture and set aside.

Apply a little bit of the mixture on the capsicum and onion. Place these on a stick along with the pork pieces.

Pre heat the Air Fryer at 290 Fahrenheit for around 5 minutes. Open the basket. Arrange the satay sticks properly. Close the basket. Keep the sticks with the pork at 180 degrees for around half an hour while the sticks with the vegetables are to be kept at the same temperature for only 7 minutes. Turn the sticks in between so that one side does not get burnt and also to provide a uniform cook.

2 cups sliced mutton

1 big capsicum (Cut this capsicum into big cubes)

1   onion (Cut it into quarters. Now separate the layers carefully.) 5 tbsp. gram flour

A pinch of salt to taste

For the filling:

2   cup fresh green coriander

½ cup mint leaves 4 tsp. fennel

2   tbsp. ginger-garlic paste 1 small onion

6-7 flakes garlic (optional) Salt to taste

3   tbsp. lemon juice

Method:

You will first need to make the chutney. Add the ingredients to a blender and make a thick paste. Slit the pieces of mutton and stuff half the paste into the cavity obtained.

Take the remaining paste and add it to the gram flour and salt. Toss the pieces of mutton in this mixture and set aside.

Apply a little bit of the mixture on the capsicum and onion. Place these on a stick along with the mutton pieces.

Pre heat the Air Fryer at 290 Fahrenheit for around 5 minutes. Open the basket. Arrange the satay sticks properly. Close the basket. Keep the sticks with the mutton at 180 degrees for around half an hour while the sticks with the vegetables are to be kept at the same temperature for only 7 minutes. Turn the sticks in between so that one side does not get burnt and also to provide a uniform cook.

35.   Chicken Wontons

Ingredients: For dough:

1 ½ cup all-purpose flour

½ tsp. salt

5 tbsp. water

For filling:

2 cups minced chicken 2 tbsp. oil

2 tsp. ginger-garlic paste 2 tsp. soya sauce

2 tsp. vinegar

Method:

Knead the dough and cover it with plastic wrap and set aside. Next, cook the ingredients for the filling and try to ensure that the chicken is covered well with the sauce.

Roll the dough and place the filling in the center. Now, wrap the dough to cover the filling and pinch the edges together.

Pre heat the Air fryer at 200° F for 5 minutes. Place the wontons in the fry basket and close it. Let them cook at the same temperature for another 20 minutes. Recommended sides are chili sauce or ketchup.

Ingredients:

36.   Beef Steak

2   lb. boneless beef cut into slices

1st Marinade:

3   tbsp. vinegar or lemon juice 2 or 3 tsp. paprika

1 tsp. black pepper 1 tsp. salt

3 tsp. ginger-garlic paste

2nd Marinade:

1 cup yogurt

4 tsp. tandoori masala

2 tbsp. dry fenugreek leaves 1 tsp. black salt

1 tsp. chat masala

1 tsp. garam masala powder 1 tsp. red chili powder

1 tsp. salt

3 drops of red color

Method:

Make the first marinade and soak the cut beef in it for four hours. While this is happening, make the second marinade and soak the beef in it overnight to let the flavors blend.

Pre heat the Air fryer at 160 degrees Fahrenheit for 5 minutes. Place the fingers in the fry basket and close it. Let them cook at the same temperature for another 15 minutes or so. Toss the fingers well so that they are cooked uniformly. Serve them with mint chutney.

37.   Chicken Samosa

Ingredients: For wrappers:

2 tbsp. unsalted butter

1 ½ cup all-purpose flour A pinch of salt to taste

Add as much water as required to make the dough stiff and firm

For filling:

1 lb. chicken (Remove the chicken from the bone and cut it into pieces)

¼ cup boiled peas

1 tsp. powdered ginger

1 or 2 green chilies that are finely chopped or mashed

½ tsp. cumin

1 tsp. coarsely crushed coriander 1 dry red chili broken into pieces A small amount of salt (to taste)

½ tsp. dried mango powder

½ tsp. red chili power. 1-2 tbsp. coriander.

Method:

You will first need to make the outer covering. In a large bowl, add the flour, butter and enough water to knead it into dough that is stiff. Transfer this to a container and leave it to rest for five minutes.

Place a pan on medium flame and add the oil. Roast the mustard seeds and once roasted, add the coriander seeds and the chopped dry red chilies. Add all the dry ingredients for the filling and mix the ingredients well. Add a little water and continue to stir the ingredients.

Make small balls out of the dough and roll them out. Cut the rolled out dough into halves and apply a little water on the edges to help you fold the halves into a cone. Add the filling to the cone and close up the samosa.

Pre-heat the Air Fryer for around 5 to 6 minutes at 300 Fahrenheit. Place all the samosas in the fry basket and close the basket properly. Keep the Air Fryer at 200 degrees for another 20 to 25 minutes. Around the halfway point, open the basket and turn the samosas over for uniform cooking. After this, fry at 250 degrees for around 10 minutes in order to give them the desired golden brown color. Serve hot. Recommended sides are tamarind or mint chutney.

1 lb. boneless fish roughly chopped 3 onions chopped

5 green chilies-roughly chopped 1 ½ tbsp. ginger paste

1 ½ tsp garlic paste 1 ½ tsp salt

3 tsp lemon juice

2 tsp garam masala

4 tbsp. chopped coriander 3 tbsp. cream

2 tbsp. coriander powder 4 tbsp. fresh mint chopped 3 tbsp. chopped capsicum 3 eggs

2 ½ tbsp. white sesame seeds

Method:

Take all the ingredients mentioned under the first heading and mix them in a bowl. Grind them thoroughly to make a smooth paste.

Take the eggs in a different bowl and beat them. Add a pinch of salt and leave them aside.

Take a flat plate and in it mix the sesame seeds and breadcrumbs.

Mold the fish mixture into small balls and flatten them into round and flat kebabs.

Dip these kebabs in the egg and salt mixture and then in the mixture of breadcrumbs and sesame seeds. Leave these kebabs in the fridge for an hour or so to set.

Pre heat the Air fryer at 160 degrees Fahrenheit for around 5 minutes. Place the kebabs in the basket and let them cook for another 25 minutes at the same temperature. Turn the kebabs over in between the cooking process to get auniform cook. Serve the kebabs with mint chutney.

½ lb. firm white fish fillet cut into fingers 1 tbsp. lemon juice

2 cups of dry breadcrumbs 1 cup oil for frying Marinade:

1   ½ tbsp. ginger-garlic paste 3 tbsp. lemon juice

2   tsp salt

1 ½ tsp pepper powder

1 tsp red chili flakes or to taste 3 eggs

5 tbsp. corn flour

2 tsp tomato ketchup

Method:

Rub a little lemon juice on the fingers and set aside. Wash the fish after an hour and pat dry. Make the marinade and transfer the fingers into the marinade. Leave them on a plate to dry for fifteen minutes. Now cover the fingers with the crumbs and set aside to dry for fifteen minutes.

Pre heat the Air Fryer at 160 degrees Fahrenheit for 5 minutes or so. Keep the fish in the fry basket now and close it properly. Let the fingers cook at the same temperature for another 25 minutes. In between the cooking process, toss the fish once in a while to avoid burning the food. Serve either with tomato ketchup or chili sauce. Mint chutney also works well with the fish.

40.   Chinese Chili

Ingredients: For chicken fingers: 1 lb. chicken (Cut into cubes) 2 ½ tsp. ginger-garlic paste

1   tsp. red chili sauce

¼ tsp. salt

¼ tsp. red chili powder/black pepper

A few drops of edible orange food coloring

For sauce:

2   tbsp. olive oil

1 ½ tsp. ginger garlic paste

½ tbsp. red chili sauce 2 tbsp. tomato ketchup 2 tsp. soya sauce

1-2 tbsp. honey

¼ tsp. Ajinomoto

1-2 tsp. red chili flakes

Method:

Mix all the ingredients for the marinade and put the chicken cubes inside and let it rest overnight.

Mix the breadcrumbs, oregano and red chili flakes well and place the marinated fingers on this mixture. Cover it with plastic wrap and leave it till right before you serve to cook.

Pre heat the Air fryer at 160 degrees Fahrenheit for 5 minutes. Place the fingers in the fry basket and close it. Let them cook at the same temperature for another 15 minutes or so. Toss the fingers well so that they are cooked uniformly.

41.   Lamb Kebab

Ingredients:

1 lb. of lamb

3 onions chopped

5 green chilies-roughly chopped 1 ½ tbsp. ginger paste

1 ½ tsp garlic paste 1 ½ tsp salt

3 tsp lemon juice

2 tsp garam masala

4 tbsp. chopped coriander 3 tbsp. cream

4 tbsp. fresh mint chopped 3 tbsp. chopped capsicum 3 eggs

2 ½ tbsp. white sesame seeds

Method:

Cut the lamb into medium sized chunks. Marinate these chunks overnight in any marinade of your choice. You can use any of the marinades mentioned in this book.

Take all the ingredients mentioned under the first heading and mix them in a bowl. Grind them thoroughly to make a smooth paste.

Take the eggs in a different bowl and beat them. Add a pinch of salt and leave them aside.

Take a flat plate and in it mix the sesame seeds and breadcrumbs.

Mold the lamb mixture into small balls and flatten them into round and flat kebabs.

Dip these kebabs in the egg and salt mixture and then in the mixture of breadcrumbs and sesame seeds. Leave these kebabs in the fridge for an hour or so to set.

Pre heat the Air fryer at 160 degrees Fahrenheit for around 5 minutes. Place the kebabs in the basket and let them cook for another 25 minutes at the same temperature. Turn the kebabs over in between the cooking process to get auniform cook. Serve the kebabs with mint chutney.

42.   Mutton Wontons

Ingredients: For dough:

1 ½ cup all-purpose flour

½ tsp. salt

5 tbsp. water

For filling:

2 cups minced mutton 2 tbsp. oil

2 tsp. ginger-garlic paste 2 tsp. soya sauce

2 tsp. vinegar

Method:

Knead the dough and cover it with plastic wrap and set aside. Next, cook the ingredients for the filling and try to ensure that the mutton is covered well with the sauce.

Roll the dough and place the filling in the center. Now, wrap the dough to cover the filling and pinch the edges together.

Pre heat the Air fryer at 200° F for 5 minutes. Place the wontons in the fry basket and close it. Let them cook at the same temperature for another 20 minutes. Recommended sides are chili sauce or ketchup.

43.   Mutton Samosa

Ingredients: For wrappers:

2 tbsp. unsalted butter

1   ½ cup all-purpose flour A pinch of salt to taste

Add as much water as required to make the dough stiff and firm

For filling:

2   cups minced mutton

¼ cup boiled peas

A small amount of ginger either grated or finely chopped 1 or 2 green chilies that are finely chopped or mashed

½ tsp cumin

1   tsp coarsely crushed whole coriander 1 dry red chili broken into pieces

A small amount of salt

½ tsp dried mango powder

½ tsp red chili power 1-2 tbsp. coriander Method:

You will first need to make the outer covering. In a large bowl, add the flour, butter and enough water to knead it into dough that is stiff. Transfer this to a container and leave it to rest for five minutes.

Place a pan on medium flame and add the oil. Roast the mustard seeds and once roasted, add the coriander seeds and the chopped dry red chilies. Add all the dry ingredients for the filling and mix the ingredients well. Add a little water and continue to stir the ingredients.

Make small balls out of the dough and roll them out. Cut the rolled out dough into halves and apply a little water on the edges to help you fold the halves into a cone. Add the filling to the cone and close up the samosa.

Pre-heat the Air Fryer for around 5 to 6 minutes at 300 Fahrenheit. Place all the samosas in the fry basket and close the basket properly. Keep the Air Fryer at 200 degrees for another 20 to 25 minutes. Around the halfway point, open the basket and turn the samosas over for uniform cooking. After this, fry at 250 degrees for around 10 minutes in order to give them the desired golden brown color. Serve hot. Recommended sides are tamarind or mint chutney.

Ingredients:

44.   Chicken Burritos

½ lb. chicken (You will need to cut the chicken into small pieces)

½ small onion chopped 1 tbsp. olive oil

2   tbsp. tomato puree

¼ tsp. red chili powder 1 tsp. of salt to taste

4-5 flour tortillas

Filling:

1 tbsp. Olive oil

1 medium onion finely sliced 3 flakes garlic crushed

1   tsp. white wine

A pinch of salt to taste

½ tsp. red chili flakes

2   carrots (Cut in to long thin slices)

Salad:

1-2 lettuce leaves shredded.

1 or 2 spring onions chopped finely. Also cut the greens.

Take one tomato. Remove the seeds and chop it into small pieces. 1 green chili chopped.

1 cup of cheddar cheese grated.

To serve:

1   cup boiled rice (not necessary).

A few flour tortillas to put the filing in.

Method:

Cook the chicken, onions and garlic in two cups of water. You will need to cook till the chicken pieces have turned very soft. Now, mash the beans very fine.

In a pan, add oil and a few more onions to the pan and cook till the onions have turned translucent. Add the tomato puree and the cooked chicken and stir. Add the chili powder and salt to the pan and continue to cook till you get athick paste. Set it aside.

For the filling, you will need to sauté the onions and garlic in oil. Add the French beans and the chopped carrots. You will need to stir-fry for a few minutes and add the remaining ingredients for the filling. Cook for another ten minutes and take the pan off the flame. Mix it well and add the

jalapenos.

To make the salad, toss the ingredients together.

Place a tortilla and add a layer of the French beans to it. Cover the edges using the chicken paste. Put the filling in the center of the tortilla along with the salad and some boiled rice. Roll up the tortilla using the chicken sauce to help you hold it together.

Pre-heat the Air Fryer for around 5 minutes at 200 Fahrenheit. Open the fry basket and keep the burritos inside. Close the basket properly. Let the Air Fryer remain at 200 Fahrenheit for another 15 minutes or so. Halfway through, remove the basket and turn all the burritos over in order to get a uniform cook. You can either serve the burritos as they are or you can cut them into pieces so that they are easier to eat. Recommended sides are salsa or some salad.

Ingredients:

45.   Lamb Cheese Sticks

2   cups lamb (Cut the lamb into long strips) 1 cup cheddar cheese

1 big lemon-juiced

1 tbsp. ginger-garlic paste

For seasoning, use salt and red chili powder in small amounts

½ tsp. carom

One or two papadums 4 or 5 tbsp. corn flour 1 cup of water
Method:

Make a mixture of lemon juice, red chili powder, salt, ginger garlic paste and carom to use as a marinade. Let the lamb pieces marinate in the mixture for some time and then roll them in dry corn flour. Leave them aside for around 20 minutes.

Take the papadum into a pan and roast them. Once they are cooked, crush them into very small pieces. Now take another container and pour around 100 ml of water into it. Dissolve 2 tbsp. of corn flour in this water. Dip the cottage cheese pieces in this solution of corn flour and roll them on to the pieces of crushed papadum so that the papadum sticks to the lamb.

Pre heat the Air Fryer for 10 minutes at 300 Fahrenheit. Then open the basket of the fryer and place the lamb pieces inside it. Close the basket properly. Let the fryer stay at 250 degrees for another 20 minutes. Halfway through, open the basket and toss the lamb around a bit to allow for uniform cooking. Once they are done, you can serve it either with ketchup or mint chutney. Another recommended side is mint chutney.

Ingredients:

46.   Tandoori Chicken

1 lb. chicken (Cut the chicken into cubes of one inch each. Make sure that they have been deboned well)

1 big capsicum (Cut this capsicum into big cubes)

1   onion (Cut it into quarters. Now separate the layers carefully.) 5 tbsp. gram flour

A pinch of salt to taste

For chutney:

2   cup fresh green coriander

½ cup mint leaves 4 tsp. fennel

2   tbsp. ginger-garlic paste 1 small onion

6-7 flakes garlic (optional) Salt to taste

3   tbsp. lemon juice

Method:

You will first need to make the chutney. Add the ingredients to a blender and make a thick paste. Slit the pieces of chicken and stuff half the paste into the cavity obtained.

Take the remaining paste and add it to the gram flour and salt. Toss the pieces of chicken in this mixture and set aside.

Apply a little bit of the mixture on the capsicum and onion. Place these on a stick along with the chicken pieces.

Pre heat the Air Fryer at 290 Fahrenheit for around 5 minutes. Open the basket. Arrange the satay sticks properly. Close the basket. Keep the sticks with the chicken at 180 degrees for around half an hour while the sticks with the vegetables are to be kept at the same temperature for only 7 minutes. Turn the sticks in between so that one side does not get burnt and also to provide a uniform cook.

47.   Prawn Wontons

Ingredients: For dough:

1 ½ cup all-purpose flour

½ tsp. salt

5 tbsp. water

For filling:

2 cups minced prawn 2 tbsp. oil

2 tsp. ginger-garlic paste 2 tsp. soya sauce

2 tsp. vinegar

Method:

Knead the dough and cover it with plastic wrap and set aside. Next, cook the ingredients for the filling and try to ensure that the prawn is covered well with the sauce.

Roll the dough and place the filling in the center. Now, wrap the dough to cover the filling and pinch the edges together.

Pre heat the Air fryer at 200° F for 5 minutes. Place the wontons in the fry basket and close it. Let them cook at the same temperature for another 20 minutes. Recommended sides are chili sauce or ketchup.

48.   Lamb Barbecue Club Sandwich

Ingredients:

2 slices of white bread 1 tbsp. softened butter

½ lb. cut lamb (Get the meat cut into cubes) 1 small capsicum

For Barbeque Sauce:

¼ tbsp. Worcestershire sauce

½ tsp. olive oil

½ flake garlic crushed

¼ cup chopped onion

½ tbsp. sugar

¼ tbsp. red chili sauce

Method:

Take the slices of bread and remove the edges. Now cut the slices horizontally.

Cook the ingredients for the sauce and wait till it thickens. Now, add the lamb to the sauce and stir till it obtains the flavors. Roast the capsicum and peel the skin off. Cut the capsicum into slices. Mix the ingredients together and apply it to the bread slices.

Pre-heat the Air Fryer for 5 minutes at 300 Fahrenheit. Open the basket of the Fryer and place the prepared sandwiches in it such that no two sandwiches are touching each other. Now keep the fryer at 250 degrees for around 15 minutes. Turn the sandwiches in between the cooking process to cook both slices. Serve the sandwiches with tomato ketchup or mint chutney.

49.   Honey Chili Chicken

Ingredients: For chicken fingers:

1 lb. chicken (Cut the chicken into slices) 2 ½ tsp. ginger-garlic paste

1   tsp. red chili sauce

¼ tsp. salt

¼ tsp. red chili powder/black pepper

A few drops of edible orange food coloring

For sauce:

2   tbsp. olive oil

1   capsicum (Cut in to long pieces)

2   small onions. Cut them into halves 1 ½ tsp. ginger garlic paste

½ tbsp. red chili sauce 2 tbsp. tomato ketchup

1   ½ tbsp. sweet chili sauce 2 tsp. soya sauce

2   tsp. vinegar

1-2 tbsp. honey

A pinch of black pepper 2 tsp. red chili flakes Method:

Create the mix for the chicken fingers and coat the chicken well with it.

Pre heat the Air fryer at 250 Fahrenheit for 5 minutes or so. Open the basket of the Fryer. Place the fingers inside the basket. Now let the fryer stay at

290 Fahrenheit for another 20 minutes. Keep tossing the fingers periodically through the cook to get auniform cook.

Add the ingredients to the sauce and cook it with the vegetables till it thickens. Add the chicken fingers to the sauce and cook till the flavors have blended.

2 slices of white bread 1 tbsp. softened butter 1 tin tuna

1 small capsicum

For Barbeque Sauce:

¼ tbsp. Worcestershire sauce

½ tsp. olive oil

¼ tsp. mustard powder

½ flake garlic crushed

¼ cup chopped onion

½ tbsp. sugar

1 tbsp. tomato ketchup

½ cup water.

¼ tbsp. red chili sauce

A pinch of salt and black pepper to taste

Method:

Take the slices of bread and remove the edges. Now cut the slices horizontally.

Cook the ingredients for the sauce and wait till it thickens. Now, add the lamb to the sauce and stir till it obtains the flavors. Roast the capsicum and peel the skin off. Cut the capsicum into slices. Mix the ingredients together and apply it to the bread slices.

Pre-heat the Air Fryer for 5 minutes at 300 Fahrenheit. Open the basket of the Fryer and place the prepared sandwiches in it such that no two sandwiches are touching each other. Now keep the fryer at 250 degrees for around 15 minutes. Turn the sandwiches in between the cooking process to cook both slices. Serve the sandwiches with tomato ketchup or mint chutney.

1   lb. boneless mutton cut into fingers 2 cup dry breadcrumbs

2   tsp. oregano

2 tsp. red chili flakes 1 cup molten cheese Marinade:

1   ½ tbsp. ginger-garlic paste 4 tbsp. lemon juice

2   tsp. salt

1 tsp. red chili powder 6 tbsp. corn flour

4 eggs

Method:

Mix all the ingredients for the marinade and put the mutton fingers inside and let it rest overnight.

Mix the breadcrumbs, oregano and red chili flakes well and place the marinated fingers on this mixture. Cover it with plastic wrap and leave it till right before you serve to cook.

Pre heat the Air fryer at 160 degrees Fahrenheit for 5 minutes. Place the fingers in the fry basket and close it. Let them cook at the same temperature for another 15 minutes or so. Toss the fingers well so that they are cooked uniformly. Serve with molten cheese.

52.   Beef Samosa

Ingredients: For wrappers:

2 tbsp. unsalted butter

1   ½ cup all-purpose flour A pinch of salt to taste

Add as much water as required to make the dough stiff and firm

For filling:

2   cups minced beef

¼ cup boiled peas

1 or 2 green chilies that are finely chopped or mashed

½ tsp cumin

1 tsp coarsely crushed whole coriander 1 dry red chili broken into pieces

A small amount of salt 1 tsp. coriander seeds Method:

You will first need to make the outer covering. In a large bowl, add the flour, butter and enough water to knead it into dough that is stiff. Transfer this to a container and leave it to rest for five minutes.

Place a pan on medium flame and add the oil. Roast the mustard seeds and once roasted, add the coriander seeds and the chopped dry red chilies. Add all the dry ingredients for the filling and mix the ingredients well. Add a little water and continue to stir the ingredients.

Make small balls out of the dough and roll them out. Cut the rolled out dough into halves and apply a little water on the edges to help you fold the halves into a cone. Add the filling to the cone and close up the samosa.

Pre-heat the Air Fryer for around 5 to 6 minutes at 300 Fahrenheit. Place all the samosas in the fry basket and close the basket properly. Keep the Air Fryer at 200 degrees for another 20 to 25 minutes. Around the halfway point, open the basket and turn the samosas over for uniform cooking. After this, fry at 250 degrees for around 10 minutes in order to give them the desired golden brown color. Serve hot. Recommended sides are tamarind or mint chutney.

Ingredients: For dough:

53.   Veal Momos

1 ½ cup all-purpose flour

½ tsp. salt

5 tbsp. water

For filling:

2 cups minced veal 2 tbsp. oil

2 tsp. ginger-garlic paste 2 tsp. soya sauce

2 tsp. vinegar

Method:

Knead the dough and cover it with plastic wrap and set aside. Next, cook the ingredients for the filling and try to ensure that the veal is covered well with the sauce.

Roll the dough and cut it into a square. Place the filling in the center. Now, wrap the dough to cover the filling and pinch the edges together.

Pre heat the Air fryer at 200° F for 5 minutes. Place the wontons in the fry basket and close it. Let them cook at the same temperature for another 20 minutes. Recommended sides are chili sauce or ketchup.

2 cups sliced veal

1 big capsicum (Cut this capsicum into big cubes)

1   onion (Cut it into quarters. Now separate the layers carefully.) 5 tbsp. gram flour

A pinch of salt to taste

For the filling:

2   cup fresh green coriander

½ cup mint leaves 4 tsp. fennel

2   tbsp. ginger-garlic paste 1 small onion

Salt to taste

3   tbsp. lemon juice

Method:

You will first need to make the chutney. Add the ingredients to a blender and make a thick paste. Slit the pieces of veal and stuff half the paste into the cavity obtained.

Take the remaining paste and add it to the gram flour and salt. Toss the pieces of veal in this mixture and set aside.

Apply a little bit of the mixture on the capsicum and onion. Place these on a stick along with the veal pieces.

Pre heat the Air Fryer at 290 Fahrenheit for around 5 minutes. Open the basket. Arrange the satay sticks properly. Close the basket. Keep the sticks with the veal at 180 degrees for around half an hour while the sticks with the vegetables are to be kept at the same temperature for only 7 minutes. Turn the sticks in between so that one side does not get burnt and also to provide a uniform cook.

2 cups sliced venison

1 big capsicum (Cut this capsicum into big cubes)

1   onion (Cut it into quarters. Now separate the layers carefully.) 5 tbsp. gram flour

A pinch of salt to taste

For the filling:

2   cup fresh green coriander

½ cup mint leaves 4 tsp. fennel

2   tbsp. ginger-garlic paste 1 small onion

6-7 flakes garlic (optional) Salt to taste

3   tbsp. lemon juice

Method:

You will first need to make the chutney. Add the ingredients to a blender and make a thick paste. Slit the pieces of venison and stuff half the paste into the cavity obtained.

Take the remaining paste and add it to the gram flour and salt. Toss the pieces of venison in this mixture and set aside.

Apply a little bit of the mixture on the capsicum and onion. Place these on a stick along with the venison pieces.

Pre heat the Air Fryer at 290 Fahrenheit for around 5 minutes. Open the basket. Arrange the satay sticks properly. Close the basket. Keep the sticks with the venison at 180 degrees for around half an hour while the sticks with the vegetables are to be kept at the same temperature for only 7 minutes. Turn the sticks in between so that one side does not get burnt and also to provide a uniform cook.

2 cups sliced quail

1 big capsicum (Cut this capsicum into big cubes)

1   onion (Cut it into quarters. Now separate the layers carefully.) 5 tbsp. gram flour

A pinch of salt to taste

For the filling:

2   cup fresh green coriander

½ cup mint leaves 4 tsp. fennel

2   tbsp. ginger-garlic paste 1 small onion

6-7 flakes garlic (optional) Salt to taste

3   tbsp. lemon juice

Method:

You will first need to make the chutney. Add the ingredients to a blender and make a thick paste. Slit the pieces of quail and stuff half the paste into the cavity obtained.

Take the remaining paste and add it to the gram flour and salt. Toss the pieces of quail in this mixture and set aside.

Apply a little bit of the mixture on the capsicum and onion. Place these on a stick along with the quail pieces.

Pre heat the Air Fryer at 290 Fahrenheit for around 5 minutes. Open the basket. Arrange the satay sticks properly. Close the basket. Keep the sticks with the quail at 180 degrees for around half an hour while the sticks with the vegetables are to be kept at the same temperature for only 7 minutes. Turn the sticks in between so that one side does not get burnt and also to provide a uniform cook.

57. Turkey Wontons

Ingredients: For dough:

1 ½ cup all-purpose flour

½ tsp. salt

5 tbsp. water

For filling:

2 cups minced turkey 2 tbsp. oil

2 tsp. ginger-garlic paste 2 tsp. soya sauce

2 tsp. vinegar

Method:

Knead the dough and cover it with plastic wrap and set aside. Next, cook the ingredients for the filling and try to ensure that the turkey is covered well with the sauce.

Roll the dough and place the filling in the center. Now, wrap the dough to cover the filling and pinch the edges together.

Pre heat the Air fryer at 200° F for 5 minutes. Place the wontons in the fry basket and close it. Let them cook at the same temperature for another 20 minutes. Recommended sides are chili sauce or ketchup.

Ingredients:

58.   Salmon Tandoor

2   lb. boneless salmon filets

1st Marinade:

3   tbsp. vinegar or lemon juice 2 or 3 tsp. paprika

1 tsp. black pepper 1 tsp. salt

3 tsp. ginger-garlic paste

2nd Marinade:

1 cup yogurt

4 tsp. tandoori masala

2 tbsp. dry fenugreek leaves 1 tsp. black salt

1 tsp. chat masala

1 tsp. garam masala powder 1 tsp. red chili powder

1 tsp. salt

3 drops of red color

Method:

Make the first marinade and soak the fileted salmon in it for four hours. While this is happening, make the second marinade and soak the salmon in it overnight to let the flavors blend.

Pre heat the Air fryer at 160 degrees Fahrenheit for 5 minutes. Place the fingers in the fry basket and close it. Let them cook at the same temperature for another 15 minutes or so. Toss the fingers well so that they are cooked uniformly. Serve them with mint chutney.

59.   Quail Samosa

Ingredients: For wrappers:

2 tbsp. unsalted butter

1 ½ cup all-purpose flour A pinch of salt to taste

Add as much water as required to make the dough stiff and firm

For filling:

1 lb. quail

¼ cup boiled peas

1 tsp. powdered ginger

1 or 2 green chilies that are finely chopped or mashed

½ tsp. cumin

1 tsp. coarsely crushed coriander 1 dry red chili broken into pieces A small amount of salt (to taste)

½ tsp. dried mango powder

½ tsp. red chili power. 1-2 tbsp. coriander.

Method:

You will first need to make the outer covering. In a large bowl, add the flour, butter and enough water to knead it into dough that is stiff. Transfer this to a container and leave it to rest for five minutes.

Place a pan on medium flame and add the oil. Roast the mustard seeds and once roasted, add the coriander seeds and the chopped dry red chilies. Add all the dry ingredients for the filling and mix the ingredients well. Add a little water and continue to stir the ingredients.

Make small balls out of the dough and roll them out. Cut the rolled out dough into halves and apply a little water on the edges to help you fold the halves into a cone. Add the filling to the cone and close up the samosa.

Pre-heat the Air Fryer for around 5 to 6 minutes at 300 Fahrenheit. Place all the samosas in the fry basket and close the basket properly. Keep the Air Fryer at 200 degrees for another 20 to 25 minutes. Around the halfway point, open the basket and turn the samosas over for uniform cooking. After this, fry at 250 degrees for around 10 minutes in order to give them the desired golden brown color. Serve hot. Recommended sides are tamarind or mint chutney.

1 lb. Carp filets

3 onions chopped

5 green chilies-roughly chopped 1 ½ tbsp. ginger paste

1 ½ tsp garlic paste 1 ½ tsp salt

3 tsp lemon juice

2 tsp garam masala

4 tbsp. chopped coriander 3 tbsp. cream

2 tbsp. coriander powder 4 tbsp. fresh mint chopped 3 tbsp. chopped capsicum 3 eggs

2 ½ tbsp. white sesame seeds

Method:

Take all the ingredients mentioned under the first heading and mix them in a bowl. Grind them thoroughly to make a smooth paste.

Take the eggs in a different bowl and beat them. Add a pinch of salt and leave them aside.

Mold the fish mixture into small balls and flatten them into round and flat Croquettes.

Dip these Croquettes in the egg and salt mixture and then in the mixture of breadcrumbs and sesame seeds. Leave these Croquettes in the fridge for an hour or so to set.

Pre heat the Air fryer at 160 degrees Fahrenheit for around 5 minutes. Place the Croquettes in the basket and let them cook for another 25 minutes at the same temperature. Turn the Croquettes over in between the cooking process to get auniform cook. Serve the Croquettes with mint chutney.

½ lb. minced turkey

½ cup breadcrumbs

A pinch of salt to taste

¼ tsp. ginger finely chopped 1 green chili finely chopped 1 tsp. lemon juice

1 tbsp. fresh coriander leaves. Chop them finely

¼ tsp. red chili powder

½ cup of boiled peas

¼ tsp. cumin powder

¼ tsp. dried mango powder

Method:

Take a container and into it pour all the masalas, onions, green chilies, peas, coriander leaves, lemon juice, ginger and 1-2 tbsp. breadcrumbs. Add the minced turkey as well. Mix all the ingredients well.

Mold the mixture into round Cutlets. Press them gently. Now roll them out carefully.

Pre heat the Air Fryer at 250 Fahrenheit for 5 minutes. Open the basket of the Fryer and arrange the Cutlets in the basket. Close it carefully. Keep the fryer at 150 degrees for around 10 or 12 minutes. In between the cooking process, turn the Cutlets over to get auniform cook. Serve hot with mint chutney.

62. Shrimp Momos

Ingredients: For dough:

1 ½ cup all-purpose flour

½ tsp. salt

5 tbsp. water

For filling:

2 cups minced shrimp 2 tbsp. oil

2 tsp. ginger-garlic paste 2 tsp. soya sauce

2 tsp. vinegar

Method:

Knead the dough and cover it with plastic wrap and set aside. Next, cook the ingredients for the filling and try to ensure that the shrimp is covered well with the sauce.

Roll the dough and cut it into a square. Place the filling in the center. Now, wrap the dough to cover the filling and pinch the edges together.

Pre heat the Air fryer at 200° F for 5 minutes. Place the wontons in the fry basket and close it. Let them cook at the same temperature for another 20 minutes. Recommended sides are chili sauce or ketchup.

1   lb. boneless salmon filets 2 cup dry breadcrumbs

2   tsp. oregano

2 tsp. red chili flakes

Marinade:

1   ½ tbsp. ginger-garlic paste 4 tbsp. lemon juice

2   tsp. salt

1 tsp. pepper powder 1 tsp. red chili powder 6 tbsp. corn flour

4 eggs

Method:

Mix all the ingredients for the marinade and put the salmon filets inside and let it rest overnight.

Mix the breadcrumbs, oregano and red chili flakes well and place the marinated fingers on this mixture. Cover it with plastic wrap and leave it till right before you serve to cook.

Pre heat the Air fryer at 160 degrees Fahrenheit for 5 minutes. Place the fingers in the fry basket and close it. Let them cook at the same temperature for another 15 minutes or so. Toss the fingers well so that they are cooked uniformly.

1   lb. boneless kangaroo 2 cup dry breadcrumbs 2 tsp. oregano

2   tsp. red chili flakes 2 tsp. garlic paste Marinade:

1   ½ tbsp. ginger-garlic paste 4 tbsp. lemon juice

2   tsp. salt

1 tsp. red chili powder 6 tbsp. corn flour

4 eggs

Method:

Mix all the ingredients for the marinade and put the kangaroo fingers inside and let it rest overnight.

Mix the breadcrumbs, oregano and red chili flakes well and place the marinated fingers on this mixture. Cover it with plastic wrap and leave it till right before you serve to cook.

Pre heat the Air fryer at 160 degrees Fahrenheit for 5 minutes. Place the fingers in the fry basket and close it. Let them cook at the same temperature for another 15 minutes or so. Toss the fingers well so that they are cooked uniformly. Drizzle the garlic paste and serve.

2 slices of white bread 1 tbsp. softened butter

½ lb. shelled oyster 1 small capsicum For Barbeque Sauce:

¼ tbsp. Worcestershire sauce

½ tsp. olive oil

½ flake garlic crushed

¼ cup chopped onion

¼ tsp. mustard powder 1 tbsp. tomato ketchup

½ tbsp. sugar

¼ tbsp. red chili sauce

½ cup water.

A pinch of salt and black pepper to taste

Method:

Take the slices of bread and remove the edges. Now cut the slices horizontally.

Cook the ingredients for the sauce and wait till it thickens. Now, add the oyster to the sauce and stir till it obtains the flavors. Roast the capsicum and peel the skin off. Cut the capsicum into slices. Mix the ingredients together and apply it to the bread slices.

Pre-heat the Air Fryer for 5 minutes at 300 Fahrenheit. Open the basket of the Fryer and place the prepared sandwiches in it such that no two sandwiches are touching each other. Now keep the fryer at 250 degrees for around 15 minutes. Turn the sandwiches in between the cooking process to cook both slices. Serve the sandwiches with tomato ketchup or mint chutney.

1   lb. quail (Cut into cubes) 2 ½ tsp. ginger-garlic paste 1 tsp. red chili sauce

¼ tsp. salt

¼ tsp. red chili powder/black pepper

A few drops of edible orange food coloring

For sauce:

2   tbsp. olive oil

1 ½ tsp. ginger garlic paste

½ tbsp. red chili sauce 2 tbsp. tomato ketchup 2 tsp. soya sauce

1-2 tbsp. honey

¼ tsp. Ajinomoto

1-2 tsp. red chili flakes

Method:

Mix all the ingredients for the marinade and put the quail cubes inside and let it rest overnight.

Mix the breadcrumbs, oregano and red chili flakes well and place the marinated fingers on this mixture. Cover it with plastic wrap and leave it till right before you serve to cook.

Pre heat the Air fryer at 160 degrees Fahrenheit for 5 minutes. Place the fingers in the fry basket and close it. Let them cook at the same temperature for another 15 minutes or so. Toss the fingers well so that they are cooked uniformly.

Ingredients:

67. Cheese Carp Fries

1 lb. carp fingers

Ingredients for the marinade:

1 tbsp. olive oil

1 tsp. mixed herbs

½ tsp. red chili flakes A pinch of salt to taste 1 tbsp. lemon juice

For the garnish:

1   cup melted cheddar cheese

Method:

Take all the ingredients mentioned under the heading "For the marinade" and mix them well.

Cook the carp fingers and soak them in the marinade.

Pre heat the Air Fryer for around 5 minutes at 300 Fahrenheit. Take out the basket of the fryer and place the carp in them. Close the basket. Now keep the fryer at 220 Fahrenheit for 20 or 25 minutes. In between the process, toss the fries twice or thrice so that they get cooked properly.

Towards the end of the cooking process (the last 2 minutes or so), sprinkle the melted cheddar cheese over the fries and serve hot.

One pizza base

Grated pizza cheese (mozzarella cheese preferably) for topping Some pizza topping sauce

Use cooking oil for brushing and topping purposes

Ingredients for topping:

2   onions chopped

2 cups mixed seafood 2 capsicums chopped

2 tomatoes that have been deseeded and chopped 1 tbsp. (optional) mushrooms/corns

2 tsp. pizza seasoning

Some cottage cheese that has been cut into small cubes (optional)

Method:

Put the pizza base in a pre-heated Air fryer for around 5 minutes. (Pre heated to 340 Fahrenheit).

Take out the base. Pour some pizza sauce on top of the base at the center. Using a spoon spread the sauce over the base making sure that you leave some gap around the circumference. Grate some mozzarella cheese and sprinkle it over the sauce layer.

Take all the vegetables and the seafood and mix them in a bowl. Add some oil and seasoning. Also add some salt and pepper according to taste. Mix them properly. Put this topping over the layer of cheese on the pizza. Now sprinkle some more grated cheese and pizza seasoning on top of this layer. Pre heat the Air Fryer at 250 Fahrenheit for around 5 minutes. Open the fry basket and place the pizza inside. Close the basket and keep the fryer at 170 degrees for another 10 minutes. If you feel that it is undercooked you may put it at the same temperature for another 2 minutes or so.

1   lb. boneless duck (Cut into fingers) 2 cup dry breadcrumbs

2   tsp. oregano

2 tsp. red chili flakes

Marinade:

1   ½ tbsp. ginger-garlic paste 4 tbsp. lemon juice

2   tsp. salt

1 tsp. pepper powder 1 tsp. red chili powder 6 tbsp. corn flour

4 eggs

Method:

Mix all the ingredients for the marinade and put the duck fingers inside and let it rest overnight.

Mix the breadcrumbs, oregano and red chili flakes well and place the marinated fingers on this mixture. Cover it with plastic wrap and leave it till right before you serve to cook.

Pre heat the Air fryer at 160 degrees Fahrenheit for 5 minutes. Place the fingers in the fry basket and close it. Let them cook at the same temperature for another 15 minutes or so. Toss the fingers well so that they are cooked uniformly.

70. Lobster Wontons

Ingredients: For dough:

1 ½ cup all-purpose flour

½ tsp. salt

5 tbsp. water

For filling:

2 cups minced lobster 2 tbsp. oil

2 tsp. ginger-garlic paste 2 tsp. soya sauce

2 tsp. vinegar

Method:

Knead the dough and cover it with plastic wrap and set aside. Next, cook the ingredients for the filling and try to ensure that the lobster is covered well with the sauce.

Roll the dough and place the filling in the center. Now, wrap the dough to cover the filling and pinch the edges together.

Pre heat the Air fryer at 200° F for 5 minutes. Place the wontons in the fry basket and close it. Let them cook at the same temperature for another 20 minutes. Recommended sides are chili sauce or ketchup.

Ingredients:

71. Seafood Platter

1 large plate with assorted prepared seafood

1st Marinade:

3 tbsp. vinegar or lemon juice 2 or 3 tsp. paprika

1 tsp. black pepper 1 tsp. salt

3 tsp. ginger-garlic paste

2nd Marinade:

1 cup yogurt

4 tsp. tandoori masala

2 tbsp. dry fenugreek leaves 1 tsp. black salt

1 tsp. chat masala

1 tsp. garam masala powder 1 tsp. red chili powder

1 tsp. salt

3 drops of red color

Method:

Make the first marinade and soak the seafood in it for four hours. While this is happening, make the second marinade and soak the seafood in it overnight to let the flavors blend.

Pre heat the Air fryer at 160 degrees Fahrenheit for 5 minutes. Place the fingers in the fry basket and close it. Let them cook at the same temperature for another 15 minutes or so. Toss the fingers well so that they are cooked uniformly. Serve them with mint chutney.

1   lb. calamari

2   ½ tsp. ginger-garlic paste 1 tsp. red chili sauce

¼ tsp. salt

¼ tsp. red chili powder/black pepper

A few drops of edible orange food coloring

For sauce:

2 tbsp. olive oil

1 ½ tsp. ginger garlic paste

½ tbsp. red chili sauce 2 tbsp. tomato ketchup 2 tsp. soya sauce

1-2 tbsp. honey

¼ tsp. Ajinomoto

1-2 tsp. red chili flakes

Method:

Mix all the ingredients for the marinade and put the calamari inside and let it rest overnight.

Mix the breadcrumbs, oregano and red chili flakes well and place the marinated fingers on this mixture. Cover it with plastic wrap and leave it till right before you serve to cook.

Pre heat the Air fryer at 160 degrees Fahrenheit for 5 minutes. Place the fingers in the fry basket and close it. Let them cook at the same temperature for another 15 minutes or so. Toss the fingers well so that they are cooked uniformly.

1 lb. minced chicken

3 tsp ginger finely chopped

1-2 tbsp. fresh coriander leaves

2 or 3 green chilies finely chopped 1 ½ tbsp. lemon juice

Salt and pepper to taste

Method:

Mix the ingredients in a clean bowl.

Mold this mixture into round and flat galettes. Wet the galettes slightly with water.

Pre heat the Air Fryer at 160 degrees Fahrenheit for 5 minutes. Place the galettes in the fry basket and let them cook for another 25 minutes at the same temperature. Keep rolling them over to get auniform cook. Serve either with mint chutney or ketchup.

1 lb. minced mutton

3 tsp ginger finely chopped

1-2 tbsp. fresh coriander leaves

2 or 3 green chilies finely chopped 1 ½ tbsp. lemon juice

Salt and pepper to taste

Method:

Mix the ingredients in a clean bowl.

Mold this mixture into round and flat galettes. Wet the galettes slightly with water.

Pre heat the Air Fryer at 160 degrees Fahrenheit for 5 minutes. Place the galettes in the fry basket and let them cook for another 25 minutes at the same temperature. Keep rolling them over to get auniform cook. Serve either with mint chutney or ketchup.

1 lb. fileted Salmon

3 tsp ginger finely chopped

1-2 tbsp. fresh coriander leaves

2 or 3 green chilies finely chopped 1 ½ tbsp. lemon juice

Salt and pepper to taste

Method:

Mix the ingredients in a clean bowl.

Mold this mixture into round and flat galettes. Wet the galettes slightly with water.

Pre heat the Air Fryer at 160 degrees Fahrenheit for 5 minutes. Place the galettes in the fry basket and let them cook for another 25 minutes at the same temperature. Keep rolling them over to get auniform cook. Serve either with mint chutney or ketchup.

1 lb. minced turkey

3 tsp ginger finely chopped

1-2 tbsp. fresh coriander leaves

2 or 3 green chilies finely chopped 1 ½ tbsp. lemon juice

Salt and pepper to taste

Method:

Mix the ingredients in a clean bowl.

Mold this mixture into round and flat galettes. Wet the galettes slightly with water.

Pre heat the Air Fryer at 160 degrees Fahrenheit for 5 minutes. Place the galettes in the fry basket and let them cook for another 25 minutes at the same temperature. Keep rolling them over to get auniform cook. Serve either with mint chutney or ketchup.

1 lb. sliced pork

3 tsp ginger finely chopped

1-2 tbsp. fresh coriander leaves

2 or 3 green chilies finely chopped 1 ½ tbsp. lemon juice

Salt and pepper to taste

Method:

Mix the ingredients in a clean bowl. Wet the galettes slightly with water.

Pre heat the Air Fryer at 160 degrees Fahrenheit for 5 minutes. Place the galettes in the fry basket and let them cook for another 25 minutes at the same temperature. Keep rolling them over to get auniform cook. Serve either with mint chutney or ketchup.

1 lb. sliced beef steak

3 tsp ginger finely chopped

1-2 tbsp. fresh coriander leaves

2 or 3 green chilies finely chopped 1 ½ tbsp. lemon juice

Salt and pepper to taste

Method:

Mix the ingredients in a clean bowl and add water to it. Make sure that the paste is not too watery but is enough to apply on the sides of the steak.

Pre heat the Air Fryer at 160 degrees Fahrenheit for 5 minutes. Place the galettes in the fry basket and let them cook for another 25 minutes at the same temperature. Keep rolling them over to get auniform cook. Serve either with mint chutney or ketchup.

1 lb. fileted carp

3 tsp ginger finely chopped

1-2 tbsp. fresh coriander leaves

2 or 3 green chilies finely chopped 1 ½ tbsp. lemon juice

Salt and pepper to taste

Method:

Mix the ingredients in a clean bowl and add water to it. Make sure that the paste is not too watery but is enough to apply on the sides of the carp filets. Pre heat the Air Fryer at 160 degrees Fahrenheit for 5 minutes. Place the galettes in the fry basket and let them cook for another 25 minutes at the same temperature. Keep rolling them over to get auniform cook. Serve either with mint chutney or ketchup.

1 lb. minced prawn

3 tsp ginger finely chopped

1-2 tbsp. fresh coriander leaves

2 or 3 green chilies finely chopped 1 ½ tbsp. lemon juice

Salt and pepper to taste

Method:

Mix the ingredients in a clean bowl.

Mold this mixture into round and flat galettes. Wet the galettes slightly with water.

Pre heat the Air Fryer at 160 degrees Fahrenheit for 5 minutes. Place the galettes in the fry basket and let them cook for another 25 minutes at the same temperature. Keep rolling them over to get auniform cook. Serve either with mint chutney or ketchup.

½ lb. sliced chicken

Method:

Put two slices together and cut them along the diagonal. In a bowl, whisk the egg whites and add some sugar.

Dip the bread triangles into this mixture. Cook the chicken now.

Pre heat the Air Fryer at 180° C for 4 minutes. Place the coated bread triangles in the fry basket and close it. Let them cook at the same temperature for another 20 minutes at least. Halfway through the process, turn the triangles over so that you get auniform cook. Top with chicken and serve.

½ lb. sliced beef

Method:

Put two slices together and cut them along the diagonal. In a bowl, whisk the egg whites and add some sugar.

Dip the bread triangles into this mixture. Cook the beef now.

Pre heat the Air Fryer at 180° C for 4 minutes. Place the coated bread triangles in the fry baskct and close it. Let them cook at the same temperature for another 20 minutes at least. Halfway through the process, turn the triangles over so that you get auniform cook. Top with beef and serve.

½ lb. sliced lamb

Method:

Put two slices together and cut them along the diagonal. In a bowl, whisk the egg whites and add some sugar.

Dip the bread triangles into this mixture. Cook the lamb now.

Pre heat the Air Fryer at 180° C for 4 minutes. Place the coated bread triangles in the fry basket and close it. Let them cook at the same temperature for another 20 minutes at least. Halfway through the process, turn the triangles over so that you get auniform cook. Top with lamb and serve.

1 cup cubed lamb

1 ½ tsp. garlic paste Salt and pepper to taste 1 tsp. dry oregano

1 tsp. dry basil

½ cup hung curd 1 tsp. lemon juice

1 tsp. red chili flakes

Method:

Add the ingredients into a separate bowl and mix them well to get aconsistent mixture.

Dip the lamb pieces in the above mixture and leave them aside for some time.

Pre heat the Air fryer at 180° C for around 5 minutes. Place the coated lamb pieces in the fry basket and close it properly. Let them cook at the same temperature for 20 more minutes. Keep turning them over in the basket so that they are cooked properly. Serve with tomato ketchup.

10 carp filets

3 onions chopped

5 green chilies-roughly chopped 1 ½ tbsp. ginger paste

1 ½ tsp. garlic paste 1 ½ tsp. salt

3 tsp. lemon juice

2 tsp. garam masala 3 eggs

2 ½ tbsp. white sesame seeds

Method:

Grind the ingredients except for the egg and form a smooth paste. Coat the filets in the paste. Now, beat the eggs and add a little salt to it.

Dip the coated filets in the egg mixture and then transfer to the sesame seeds and coat the florets well. Place the vegetables on a stick.

Pre heat the Air fryer at 160 degrees Fahrenheit for around 5 minutes. Place the sticks in the basket and let them cook for another 25 minutes at the same temperature. Turn the sticks over in between the cooking process to get auniform cook.

1 cup cubed duck

1 ½ tsp. garlic paste Salt and pepper to taste 1 tsp. dry oregano

1 tsp. dry basil

½ cup hung curd 1 tsp. lemon juice

1 tsp. red chili flakes

Method:

Add the ingredients into a separate bowl and mix them well to get aconsistent mixture.

Dip the duck pieces in the above mixture and leave them aside for some time.

Pre heat the Air fryer at 180° C for around 5 minutes. Place the coated duck pieces in the fry basket and close it properly. Let them cook at the same temperature for 20 more minutes. Keep turning them over in the basket so that they are cooked properly. Serve with tomato ketchup.

1   lb.   boneless   caribou   cut   into   fingers   2   cup   dry breadcrumbs

2   tsp. oregano

2 tsp. red chili flakes

Marinade:

1   ½ tbsp. ginger-garlic paste 4 tbsp. lemon juice

2   tsp. salt

1 tsp. pepper powder 1 tsp. red chili powder 6 tbsp. corn flour

4 eggs

Method:

Mix all the ingredients for the marinade and put the caribou fingers inside and let it rest overnight.

Mix the breadcrumbs, oregano and red chili flakes well and place the marinated fingers on this mixture. Cover it with plastic wrap and leave it till right before you serve to cook.

Pre heat the Air fryer at 160 degrees Fahrenheit for 5 minutes. Place the fingers in the fry basket and close it. Let them cook at the same temperature for another 15 minutes or so. Toss the fingers well so that they are cooked uniformly.

6 slices bacon

2 cup dry breadcrumbs 2 tsp. oregano

2 tsp. red chili flakes 2 tsp. garlic paste Marinade:

1   ½ tbsp. ginger-garlic paste 4 tbsp. lemon juice

2   tsp. salt

1 tsp. red chili powder 6 tbsp. corn flour

4 eggs

Method:

Mix all the ingredients for the marinade and put the bacon slices inside and let it rest overnight.

Mix the breadcrumbs, oregano and red chili flakes well and place the marinated fingers on this mixture. Cover it with plastic wrap and leave it till right before you serve to cook.

Pre heat the Air fryer at 160 degrees Fahrenheit for 5 minutes. Place the fingers in the fry basket and close it. Let them cook at the same temperature for another 15 minutes or so. Toss the fingers well so that they are cooked uniformly. Drizzle the garlic paste and serve.

2 slices of white bread 1 tbsp. softened butter 1 lb. ham (Sliced)

1 small capsicum

For Barbeque Sauce:

¼ tbsp. Worcestershire sauce

½ tsp. olive oil

½ flake garlic crushed

¼ tsp. mustard powder

¼ cup chopped onion

½ tbsp. sugar

1 tbsp. tomato ketchup

¼ tbsp. red chili sauce

½ cup water.

A pinch of salt and black pepper to taste

Method:

Take the slices of bread and remove the edges. Now cut the slices horizontally.

Cook the ingredients for the sauce and wait till it thickens. Now, add the ham slices to the sauce and stir till it obtains the flavors. Roast the capsicum and peel the skin off. Cut the capsicum into slices. Mix the ingredients together and apply it to the bread slices.

Pre-heat the Air Fryer for 5 minutes at 300 Fahrenheit. Open the basket of the Fryer and place the prepared sandwiches in it such that no two sandwiches are touching each other. Now keep the fryer at 250 degrees for around 15 minutes. Turn the sandwiches in between the cooking process to cook both slices. Serve the sandwiches with tomato ketchup or mint chutney.

1   lb. cubed pheasant

2   ½ tsp. ginger-garlic paste 1 tsp. red chili sauce

¼ tsp. salt

¼ tsp. red chili powder/black pepper

A few drops of edible orange food coloring

For sauce:

2 tbsp. olive oil

1 ½ tsp. ginger garlic paste

½ tbsp. red chili sauce 2 tbsp. tomato ketchup 2 tsp. soya sauce

1-2 tbsp. honey

¼ tsp. Ajinomoto

1-2 tsp. red chili flakes

Method:

Mix all the ingredients for the marinade and put the pheasant cubes inside and let it rest overnight.

Mix the breadcrumbs, oregano and red chili flakes well and place the marinated fingers on this mixture. Cover it with plastic wrap and leave it till right before you serve to cook.

Pre heat the Air fryer at 160 degrees Fahrenheit for 5 minutes. Place the fingers in the fry basket and close it. Let them cook at the same temperature for another 15 minutes or so. Toss the fingers well so that they are cooked uniformly.

Ingredients:

91. Duck Liver fries

1 lb. duck liver (Cut in to long fingers)

Ingredients for the marinade:

1 tbsp. olive oil

1 tsp. mixed herbs

½ tsp. red chili flakes A pinch of salt to taste 1 tbsp. lemon juice

For the garnish:

1 cup melted cheddar cheese

Method:

Take all the ingredients mentioned under the heading "For the marinade" and mix them well.

Cook the duck liver fingers and soak them in the marinade.

Pre heat the Air Fryer for around 5 minutes at 300 Fahrenheit. Take out the basket of the fryer and place the chicken fingers in them. Close the basket. Now keep the fryer at 220 Fahrenheit for 20 or 25 minutes. In between the process, toss the fries twice or thrice so that they get cooked properly.

Towards the end of the cooking process (the last 2 minutes or so), sprinkle the cut coriander leaves on the fries. Add the melted cheddar cheese over the fries and serve hot.

1 lb. thinly sliced ham

3 tsp ginger finely chopped

1-2 tbsp. fresh coriander leaves

2 or 3 green chilies finely chopped 1 ½ tbsp. lemon juice

Salt and pepper to taste

Method:

Mix the ingredients in a clean bowl and add water to it. Make sure that the paste is not too watery but is enough to apply on the sides of the ham slices. Pre heat the Air Fryer at 160 degrees Fahrenheit for 5 minutes. Place the galettes in the fry basket and let them cook for another 25 minutes at the same temperature. Keep rolling them over to get auniform cook. Serve either with mint chutney or ketchup.

1 lb. minced clam

3 tsp ginger finely chopped

1-2 tbsp. fresh coriander leaves

2 or 3 green chilies finely chopped 1 ½ tbsp. lemon juice

Salt and pepper to taste

Method:

Mix the ingredients in a clean bowl.

Mold this mixture into round and flat galettes. Wet the galettes slightly with water.

Pre heat the Air Fryer at 160 degrees Fahrenheit for 5 minutes. Place the galettes in the fry basket and let them cook for another 25 minutes at the same temperature. Keep rolling them over to get auniform cook. Serve either with mint chutney or ketchup.

Bread slices (brown or white) 1 egg white for every 2 slices 1 tsp sugar for every 2 slices

½ lb. sliced ham

Method:

Put two slices together and cut them along the diagonal. In a bowl, whisk the egg whites and add some sugar.

Dip the bread triangles into this mixture. Cook the chicken now.

Pre heat the Air Fryer at 180° C for 4 minutes. Place the coated bread triangles in the fry basket and close it. Let them cook at the same temperature for another 20 minutes at least. Halfway through the process, turn the triangles over so that you get auniform cook. Top with ham and serve.

2 cups sliced pheasant

1 big capsicum (Cut this capsicum into big cubes)

1   onion (Cut it into quarters. Now separate the layers carefully.) 5 tbsp. gram flour

A pinch of salt to taste

For the filling:

2   cup fresh green coriander

½ cup mint leaves 4 tsp. fennel

2   tbsp. ginger-garlic paste 1 small onion

6-7 flakes garlic (optional) Salt to taste

3   tbsp. lemon juice

Method:

You will first need to make the chutney. Add the ingredients to a blender and make a thick paste. Slit the pieces of pheasant and stuff half the paste into the cavity obtained.

Take the remaining paste and add it to the gram flour and salt. Toss the pieces of pheasant in this mixture and set aside.

Apply a little bit of the mixture on the capsicum and onion. Place these on a stick along with the pheasant pieces.

Pre heat the Air Fryer at 290 Fahrenheit for around 5 minutes. Open the basket. Arrange the satay sticks properly. Close the basket. Keep the sticks with the mutton at 180 degrees for around half an hour while the sticks with the vegetables are to be kept at the same temperature for only 7 minutes. Turn the sticks in between so that one side does not get burnt and also to provide a uniform cook.

96. Seafood Wontons

Ingredients: For dough:

1 ½ cup all-purpose flour

½ tsp. salt

5 tbsp. water

For filling:

2 cups minced seafood (prawns, shrimp, oysters, scallops) 2 tbsp. oil

2 tsp. ginger-garlic paste 2 tsp. soya sauce

2 tsp. vinegar

Method:

Knead the dough and cover it with plastic wrap and set aside. Next, cook the ingredients for the filling and try to ensure that the seafood is covered well with the sauce.

Roll the dough and place the filling in the center. Now, wrap the dough to cover the filling and pinch the edges together.

Pre heat the Air fryer at 200° F for 5 minutes. Place the wontons in the fry basket and close it. Let them cook at the same temperature for another 20 minutes. Recommended sides are chili sauce or ketchup.

Ingredients:

97.   Squab Cutlet

2   lb. boneless squab cut into slices

1st Marinade:

3   tbsp. vinegar or lemon juice 2 or 3 tsp. paprika

1 tsp. black pepper 1 tsp. salt

3 tsp. ginger-garlic paste

2nd Marinade:

1 cup yogurt

4 tsp. tandoori masala

2 tbsp. dry fenugreek leaves 1 tsp. black salt

1 tsp. chat masala

1 tsp. garam masala powder 1 tsp. red chili powder

1 tsp. salt

3 drops of red color

Method:

Make the first marinade and soak the cut squab in it for four hours. While this is happening, make the second marinade and soak the squab in it overnight to let the flavors blend.

Pre heat the Air fryer at 160 degrees Fahrenheit for 5 minutes. Place the fingers in the fry basket and close it. Let them cook at the same temperature for another 15 minutes or so. Toss the fingers well so that they are cooked uniformly. Serve them with mint chutney.

98.   Poultry Samosa

Ingredients: For wrappers:

2 tbsp. unsalted butter

1 ½ cup all-purpose flour A pinch of salt to taste Water to knead the dough For filling:

1 lb. mixed minced poultry (squab, chicken, duck, pheasant, turkey)

¼ cup boiled peas

1 tsp. powdered ginger

1 or 2 green chilies that are finely chopped or mashed

½ tsp. cumin

1 tsp. coarsely crushed coriander 1 dry red chili broken into pieces A small amount of salt (to taste)

½ tsp. dried mango powder

½ tsp. red chili power. 1-2 tbsp. coriander.

Method:

You will first need to make the outer covering. In a large bowl, add the flour, butter and enough water to knead it into dough that is stiff. Transfer this to a container and leave it to rest for five minutes.

Place a pan on medium flame and add the oil. Roast the mustard seeds and once roasted, add the coriander seeds and the chopped dry red chilies. Add all the dry ingredients for the filling and mix the ingredients well. Add a little water and continue to stir the ingredients.

Make small balls out of the dough and roll them out. Cut the rolled out dough into halves and apply a little water on the edges to help you fold the halves into a cone. Add the filling to the cone and close up the samosa.

Pre-heat the Air Fryer for around 5 to 6 minutes at 300 Fahrenheit. Place all the samosas in the fry basket and close the basket properly. Keep the Air Fryer at 200 degrees for another 20 to 25 minutes. Around the halfway point, open the basket and turn the samosas over for uniform cooking. After this, fry at 250 degrees for around 10 minutes in order to give them the desired golden brown color. Serve hot. Recommended sides are tamarind or mint chutney.

1 lb. lobster (Shelled and cubed) 3 onions chopped

5 green chilies-roughly chopped 1 ½ tbsp. ginger paste

1 ½ tsp garlic paste 1 ½ tsp salt

3 tsp lemon juice

2 tsp garam masala

4 tbsp. chopped coriander 3 tbsp. cream

2 tbsp. coriander powder 4 tbsp. fresh mint chopped 3 tbsp. chopped capsicum 3 eggs

2 ½ tbsp. white sesame seeds

Method:

Take all the ingredients mentioned under the first heading and mix them in a bowl. Grind them thoroughly to make a smooth paste.

Take the eggs in a different bowl and beat them. Add a pinch of salt and leave them aside.

Take a flat plate and in it mix the sesame seeds and breadcrumbs.

Dip the lobster cubes in the egg and salt mixture and then in the mixture of breadcrumbs and sesame seeds. Leave these kebabs in the fridge for an hour or so to set.

Pre heat the Air fryer at 160 degrees Fahrenheit for around 5 minutes. Place the kebabs in the basket and let them cook for another 25 minutes at the same temperature. Turn the kebabs over in between the cooking process to get auniform cook. Serve the kebabs with mint chutney.

½ lb. squab fingers

2 cups of dry breadcrumbs 1 cup oil for frying Marinade:

1   ½ tbsp. ginger-garlic paste 3 tbsp. lemon juice

2   tsp salt

1 ½ tsp pepper powder

1 tsp red chili flakes or to taste 3 eggs

5 tbsp. corn flour

2 tsp tomato ketchup

Method:

Make the marinade and transfer the fingers into the marinade. Leave them on a plate to dry for fifteen minutes. Now cover the fingers with the crumbs and set aside to dry for fifteen minutes.

Pre heat the Air Fryer at 160 degrees Fahrenheit for 5 minutes or so. Keep the fish in the fry basket now and close it properly. Let the fingers cook at the same temperature for another 25 minutes. In between the cooking process, toss the fish once in a while to avoid burning the food. Serve either with tomato ketchup or chili sauce. Mint chutney also works well with the fish.

Chapter 2: Desserts and Sweets

1 ½ cup plain flour

3 tbsp. unsalted butter 2 tbsp. powdered sugar 2 cups cold water Filling:

2   cups sliced strawberries 1 cup fresh cream

3   tbsp. butter

Method:

In a large bowl, mix the flour, cocoa powder, butter and sugar with your fingers. The mixture should resemble breadcrumbs. Knead the dough using the cold milk and wrap it and leave it to cool for ten minutes. Roll the dough out into the pie and prick the sides of the pie.

Mix the ingredients for the filling in a bowl. Make sure that it is a little thick.

Preheat the fryer to 300 Fahrenheit for five minutes. You will need to place the tin in the basket and cover it. When the pastry has turned golden brown, you will need to remove the tin and let it cool. Cut into slices and serve with a dollop of cream.

1   cup strawberry juice 2 cups milk

2   tbsp. custard powder 3 tbsp. powdered sugar 3 tbsp. unsalted butter 1 cup strawberry slices

Method:

Boil the milk and the sugar in a pan and add the custard powder followed by the strawberry juice and stir till you get athick mixture.

Preheat the fryer to 300 Fahrenheit for five minutes. Place the dish in the basket and reduce the temperature to 250 Fahrenheit. Cook for ten minutes and set aside to cool. Garnish with strawberry.

1   cup banana juice 2 cups milk

2   tbsp. custard powder 3 tbsp. powdered sugar 3 tbsp. unsalted butter

3   tbsp. chopped mixed nuts

Method:

Boil the milk and the sugar in a pan and add the custard powder followed by the banana juice and stir till you get athick mixture.

Preheat the fryer to 300 Fahrenheit for five minutes. Place the dish in the basket and reduce the temperature to 250 Fahrenheit. Cook for ten minutes and set aside to cool. Garnish with nuts.

2 cups almond powder 2 cups milk

1   tsp. gelatin

2   tbsp. custard powder 3 tbsp. powdered sugar 3 tbsp. unsalted butter

Method:

Boil the milk and the sugar in a pan and add the custard powder followed by the almond powder and stir till you get athick mixture. Add the gelatin and mix the ingredients well.

Preheat the fryer to 300 Fahrenheit for five minutes. Place the dish in the basket and reduce the temperature to 250 Fahrenheit. Cook for ten minutes and set aside to cool.

1   cup coconut milk 1 cup almond flour 2 cups milk

2   tbsp. custard powder 3 tbsp. powdered sugar 3 tbsp. unsalted butter Method:

Boil the milk and the sugar in a pan and add the custard powder followed by the flour and coconut milk and stir till you get athick mixture.

Preheat the fryer to 300 Fahrenheit for five minutes. Place the dish in the basket and reduce the temperature to 250 Fahrenheit. Cook for ten minutes and set aside to cool.

2 cups milk

2 cups custard powder 3 tbsp. powdered sugar 3 tbsp. unsalted butter 4 tbsp. caramel

Method:

Boil the milk and the sugar in a pan and add the custard powder and stir till you get athick mixture.

Preheat the fryer to 300 Fahrenheit for five minutes. Place the dish in the basket and reduce the temperature to 250 Fahrenheit. Cook for ten minutes and set aside to cool.

Spread the caramel over the dish and serve warm.

1 orange (zested)

1 ½ cups almond flour 3 eggs

1   tbsp. honey

2   tsp. dried basil

2 tsp. dried parsley Salt and Pepper to taste 3 tbsp. Butter

Method:

Preheat the air fryer to 250 Fahrenheit.

In a small bowl, mix the ingredients together. Ensure that the mixture is smooth and well balanced.

Take a pancake mold and grease it with butter. Add the batter to the mold and place it in the air fryer basket.

Cook till both the sides of the pancake have browned on both sides and serve with maple syrup.

2 cups milk

2 cups almond flour

2 tbsp. custard powder 3 tbsp. powdered sugar 3 tbsp. unsalted butter 2 cups figs

Method:

Boil the milk and the sugar in a pan and add the custard powder followed by the almond flour and stir till you get athick mixture. Chop the figs fine and add it to the mixture.

Preheat the fryer to 300 Fahrenheit for five minutes. Place the dish in the basket and reduce the temperature to 250 Fahrenheit. Cook for ten minutes and set aside to cool.

2 cups almond flour 2 cups milk

2 tbsp. custard powder 3 tbsp. powdered sugar 3 tbsp. unsalted butter 2 cups apricot

Method:

Boil the milk and the sugar in a pan and add the custard powder followed by the almond powder and stir till you get athick mixture. Chop the apricot finely and add to the mixture.

Preheat the fryer to 300 Fahrenheit for five minutes. Place the dish in the basket and reduce the temperature to 250 Fahrenheit. Cook for ten minutes and set aside to cool.

Spread the fruits on the bread and serve.

10. Baked Cream

Ingredients: For the cream: 2 cups condensed milk 2 cups fresh cream

For garnishing:

1 cup fresh strawberries 1 cup fresh blueberries 1 cup blackberries Handful of mint leaves 3 tsp. sugar

4 tsp. water

Method:

Blend the cream and add the milk to it. Whisk the ingredients well together and transfer this mixture into small baking bowls ensuring you do not overfill the bowls.

Preheat the fryer to 300 Fahrenheit for five minutes. You will need to place the bowls in the basket and cover it. Cook it for fifteen minutes. When you shake the bowls, the mixture should just shake but not break.

Leave it in the refrigerator to set and then arrange the fruits, garnish and serve.

2 cups finely chopped pistachio

Method:

Boil the milk and the sugar in a pan and add the custard powder followed by the almond flour and stir till you get a thick mixture. Add the pistachio nuts to the mixture.

Preheat the fryer to 300 Fahrenheit for five minutes. Place the dish in the basket and reduce the temperature to 250 Fahrenheit. Cook for ten minutes and set aside to cool.

2 oranges (sliced)

2 persimmons (sliced)

Method:

Boil the milk and the sugar in a pan and add the custard powder followed by the almond flour and stir till you get a thick mixture. Add the sliced fruits to the mixture.

Preheat the fryer to 300 Fahrenheit for five minutes. Place the dish in the basket and reduce the temperature to 250 Fahrenheit. Cook for ten minutes and set aside to cool.

1   cup blueberry juice 2 cups milk

2   tbsp. custard powder 3 tbsp. powdered sugar 3 tbsp. unsalted butter Method:

Boil the milk and the sugar in a pan and add the custard powder followed by the blueberry juice and stir till you get athick mixture.

Preheat the fryer to 300 Fahrenheit for five minutes. Place the dish in the basket and reduce the temperature to 250 Fahrenheit. Cook for ten minutes and set aside to cool.

2 cups coconut milk 1 cup fresh cream

2 tbsp. custard powder 3 tbsp. powdered sugar 3 tbsp. unsalted butter 1 cup pineapple slices 1 cup mango slices

1 cup banana slices

Method:

Boil the milk and the sugar in a pan and add the custard powder followed by the coconut milk and fresh cream and stir till you get athick mixture. Add the sliced fruits to the mixture.

Preheat the fryer to 300 Fahrenheit for five minutes. Place the dish in the basket and reduce the temperature to 250 Fahrenheit. Cook for ten minutes and set aside to cool.

1   ½ cups almond flour 3 eggs

2   tsp. dried basil

2 tsp. dried parsley Salt and Pepper to taste 3 tbsp. Butter

Method:

Preheat the air fryer to 250 Fahrenheit.

In a small bowl, mix the ingredients together. Ensure that the mixture is smooth and well balanced.

Take a pancake mold and grease it with butter. Add the batter to the mold and place it in the air fryer basket. Cook till both the sides of the pancake have browned on both sides and serve with maple syrup.

2   tbsp. custard powder 3 tbsp. powdered sugar 2 tbsp. rice

3   tbsp. unsalted butter

Method:

Boil the milk and the sugar in a pan and add the custard powder and stir till you get athick mixture. Add the rice to the bowl and ensure that the mixture becomes slightly thicker.

Preheat the fryer to 300 Fahrenheit for five minutes. Place the dish in the basket and reduce the temperature to 250 Fahrenheit. Cook for ten minutes and set aside to cool.

2 cups soaked sagu

2 tbsp. custard powder 3 tbsp. powdered sugar 3 tbsp. unsalted butter Method:

Boil the milk and the sugar in a pan and add the custard powder followed by the sagu and stir till you get athick mixture.

Preheat the fryer to 300 Fahrenheit for five minutes. Place the dish in the basket and reduce the temperature to 250 Fahrenheit. Cook for ten minutes and set aside to cool.

2 cups All-purpose flour 1 ½ cup milk

1   tbsp. cardamom powder

½ tsp. baking powder

½ tsp. baking soda 2 tbsp. butter

2   tbsp. sugar Muffin cups Method:

Mix the ingredients together and use your fingers to get acrumbly mixture. Add the baking soda and the vinegar to the milk and mix continuously. Add this milk to the mixture and create a batter, which you will need to transfer to the muffin cups.

Preheat the fryer to 300 Fahrenheit for five minutes. You will need to place the muffin cups in the basket and cover it. Cook the muffins for fifteen minutes and check whether or not the muffins are cooked using a toothpick. Remove the cups and serve hot.

2   cups minced cranberry 1 ½ cups almond flour

3   eggs

2 tsp. dried basil

2 tsp. dried parsley Salt and Pepper to taste 3 tbsp. Butter

Method:

Preheat the air fryer to 250 Fahrenheit.

In a small bowl, mix the ingredients together. Ensure that the mixture is smooth and well balanced.

Take a pancake mold and grease it with butter. Add the batter to the mold and place it in the air fryer basket. Cook till both the sides of the pancake have browned on both sides and serve with maple syrup.

2 cups milk

2 cups almond flour

1 tbsp. vanilla essence 2 tbsp. custard powder 3 tbsp. powdered sugar 3 tbsp. unsalted butter Method:

Boil the milk and the sugar in a pan and add the custard powder followed by the almond flour and the vanilla essence and stir till you get athick mixture.

Preheat the fryer to 300 Fahrenheit for five minutes. Place the dish in the basket and reduce the temperature to 250 Fahrenheit. Cook for ten minutes and set aside to cool.

3 cups cocoa powder 3 eggs

2 tsp. dried basil

2 tsp. dried parsley Salt and Pepper to taste 3 tbsp. Butter

1   cup chocolate chips

Method:

Preheat the air fryer to 250 Fahrenheit.

In a small bowl, mix the ingredients, except for the chocolate chips, together. Ensure that the mixture is smooth and well balanced.

Take a waffle mold and grease it with butter. Add the batter to the mold and place it in the air fryer basket. Cook till both the sides have browned. Garnish with chips and serve.

2   cups milk

2 tbsp. saffron

2 cups almond flour

2 tbsp. custard powder 3 tbsp. powdered sugar 3 tbsp. unsalted butter Method:

Boil the milk and the sugar in a pan and add the custard powder followed by the almond flour and stir till you get athick mixture. Mix the saffron into the mixture and stir till the color has spread well.

Preheat the fryer to 300 Fahrenheit for five minutes. Place the dish in the basket and reduce the temperature to 250 Fahrenheit. Cook for ten minutes and set aside to cool.

2 zucchinis (shredded) 1 ½ cups almond flour 3 eggs

2 tsp. dried basil

2 tsp. dried parsley Salt and Pepper to taste 3 tbsp. Butter

Method:

Preheat the air fryer to 250 Fahrenheit.

In a small bowl, mix the ingredients together. Ensure that the mixture is smooth and well balanced.

Take a pancake mold and grease it with butter. Add the batter to the mold and place it in the air fryer basket.

Cook till both the sides of the pancake have browned on both sides and serve with maple syrup.

24. An Upside Down Pineapple cake

Ingredients: For the batter:

2 tbsp. butter (Preferably unsalted butter)

¼ cup condensed milk 2 tsp. pineapple essence

2 cups All Purpose Flour (You will need to split the flour into two parts – 1

½ cup and another ½ cup)

¼ tsp. baking powder

¼ tsp. baking soda

Edible yellow food coloring

½ cup drinking soda

½ tbsp. powdered sugar

For the tin preparation:

6 slices pineapple

3 tbsp. sugar (This is to make the caramel) 8 cherries

Method:

You will first need to prepare the tin. Grease the tin with butter and line it on all sides with the butter paper. You will now have to dust the tin with the flour. Add the slices of the pineapple to the base of the tin followed by the cherries. You will need to cut the cherries into halves and place it on the cavities.

You will now have to melt the sugar and make it into a caramel. Pour this caramel into the tin and set it aside.

Take a large mixing bowl and add the ingredients for the batter. You will need to first sieve the flour, baking soda and powder and then add them to the bowl. Now, add the butter to the bowl and beat the ingredients. Add the sugar and the condensed milk to the bowl and beat till you get auniform mixture. Add the essence and the yellow coloring followed by the dry ingredients to the bowl. Make sure that there are no lumps in the batter. Transfer the batter into the tin.

Preheat the fryer to 300 Fahrenheit for five minutes. You will need to place the tin in the basket and cover it. Cook the cake for fifteen minutes and check whether or not the cake is cooked using a toothpick. Remove the tin and cut the cake into slices and serve.

1 ½ cup plain flour

½ cup cocoa powder 3 tbsp. unsalted butter

2 tbsp. powdered sugar 2 cups cold water

1 tbsp. sliced cashew

For Truffle filling:

1 ½ melted chocolate 1 cup fresh cream

3 tbsp. butter

Method:

In a large bowl, mix the flour, cocoa powder, butter and sugar with your fingers. The mixture should resemble breadcrumbs. Knead the dough using the cold milk and wrap it and leave it to cool for ten minutes. Roll the dough out into the pie and prick the sides of the pie.

Mix the ingredients for the filling in a bowl. Make sure that it is a little thick. Add the filling to the pie and cover it with the second round.

Preheat the fryer to 300 Fahrenheit for five minutes. You will need to place the tin in the basket and cover it. When the pastry has turned golden brown, you will need to remove the tin and let it cool. Cut into slices and serve with a dollop of cream.

CPSIA information can be obtained
at www.ICGtesting.com
Printed in the USA
BVHW072012240621
610373BV00001B/21